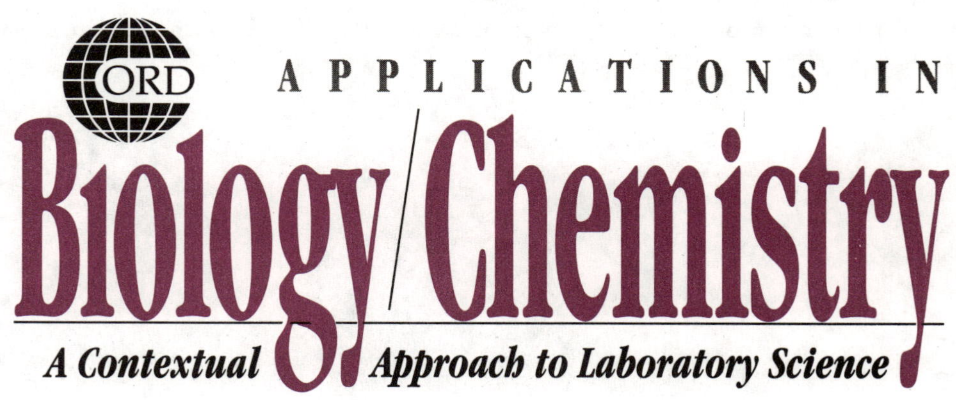

Water

Developed by the Center for Occupational Research and Development and sponsored by a consortium of State Vocational Education Agencies with the cooperation and support of science educators.

Appreciation is expressed to Alan Kousen, text consultant, to Carolyn Prescott and Woody Baker for text contributions, and to Woody Baker, Alan Kousen, and Jim Cockerill for help in lab development.

Editorial Staff:
Woody Baker
James Cockerill
Carolyn Prescott
Bonnie Rinard

Published and distributed by:
CORD Communications
324 Kelly Drive
Waco, Texas 76710
817-776-1822 FAX 817-776-3906

Printed in USA December 93

ISBN 1-55502-363-0 (Applied Biology/Chemistry)
ISBN 1-55502-400-9 (Water)

Preface

Have you ever had the water turned off for an hour or two while a plumber was at work? You got ready to take a shower, only to realize . . . That's okay, you think, I'll just have breakfast first, let me boil this egg . . . only to realize again. No problem, you say, I'll just get a load of clothes in the washer and eat breakfast out, only the washer, of course, requires water. In fact, a great many of our daily activities require water and many of the things we do for fun require water, too.

Swimming, bathing, washing your hair, brushing your teeth, cleaning your clothes, boiling an egg, making a soup, water skiing, washing your face, watering a garden, boating, washing the car, showering, washing the dishes, diving, making iced tea—the list of all the ways you use water goes on and on.

Water is used in many other ways that we don't see. Generating electricity? It takes water, and lots of it. How about food and household products? Soy sauce, canned soups, dishwashing liquid, moisturizing lotion—all contain water. It takes a lot of water to grow the food we eat. Water is used to manufacture a lot of the products we use every day.

Water is so essential to life that it is distressing to hear about problems of water quality or water quantity. And you are part of a generation that has grown up hearing about water problems. Water pollution is a term you probably first heard in kindergarten. Now you are old enough that you need to sort out what you hear about water quality and figure out your own responsibility for wisely using water.

However, most of this unit isn't about water problems. It's about how water behaves and what it can do. You'll learn about how water supports life and how it is used in industry and agriculture. Water's amazing properties—its polarity, its heat capacity and its ability to act as a solvent—make it useful in a thousand different ways. Only by understanding what water can do and how it's used can you begin to sort out questions about how well we are taking care of our water.

Table of Contents

Water

UNIT GOALS

After you complete this unit, you will be able to—

1. Evaluate the effect of different water uses on water quality and water quantity.
2. Analyze the role of water in maintaining life: as a transporter of nutrients, in biochemical reactions, in maintaining water balance and in regulating temperature.
3. Express the concentration of solutes in a solvent appropriately according to the occupational context.
4. Carry out titration procedures such as might be used in an occupational setting.
5. Analyze neutralization reactions and reactions involving buffer solutions such as those that might be carried out in an industrial setting.
6. Interpret pH readings and use the pH scale as an indicator of waters acidity or alkalinity.
7. Explain tests to determine water quality, including pH, biochemical oxygen demand, total solids, and concentrations of various solutes in water.
8. Link water-treatment methods to different types of wastewater contamination that treatment is intended to address.
9. Suggest several different methods to prevent water pollution during personal or domestic use of water and handling of wastes.

SUBUNIT 1

Why Is Water Important?

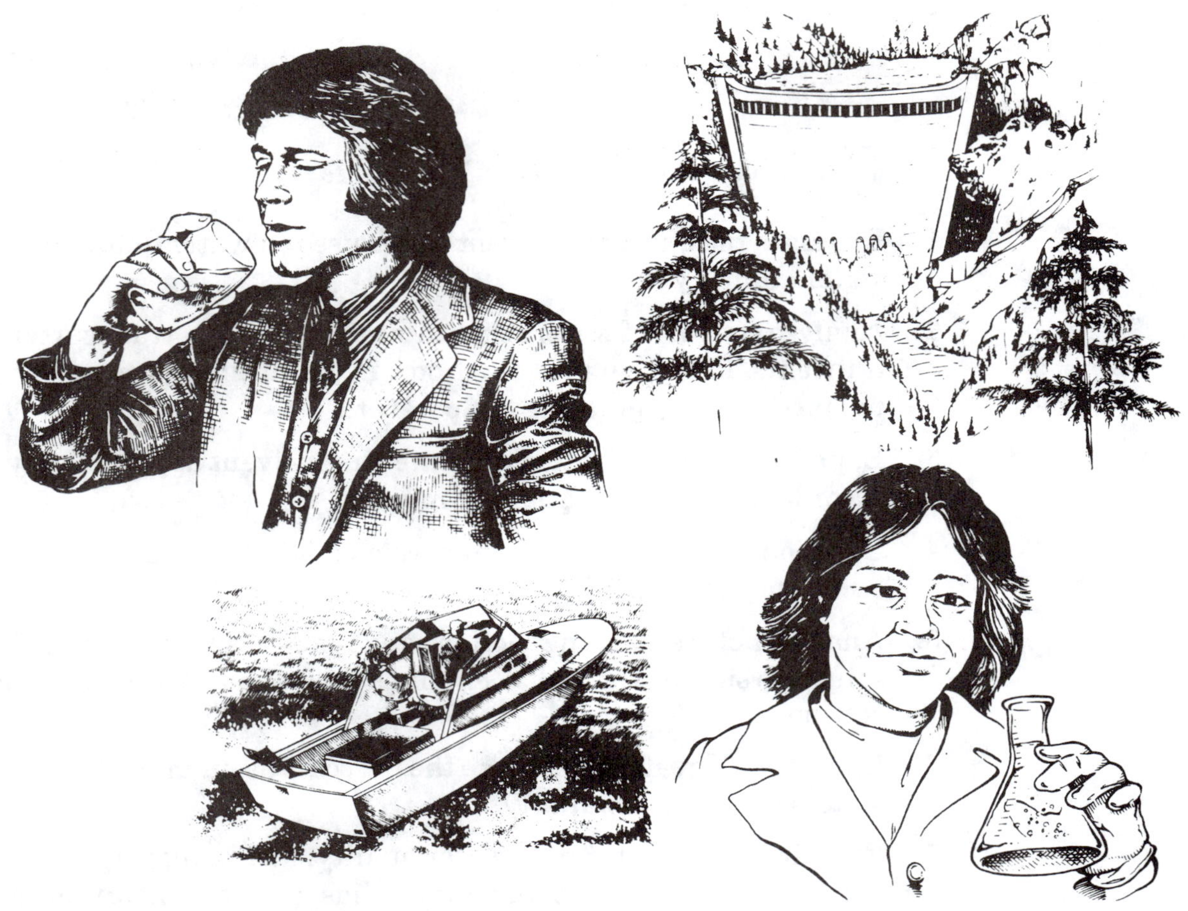

THINK ABOUT IT

- Describe the way that water is used in each instance above.
- Can you think of another liquid that would substitute for water in each instance? Why?
- What is unique about water?
- What makes it useful?

SUBUNIT OBJECTIVES

After you complete this subunit, you will be able to —

1. Investigate the sources and uses of water in your community.
2. Categorize water uses based on the properties of water.
3. Explain how water is used in a home heating system, a power plant condenser, an evaporative cooler, and a car radiator.
4. Compare three types of mixtures involving water and other substances.
5. Explain why water represents such an important habitat for organisms.
6. Devise a rule to predict whether a material will float in water.
7. Investigate the structure of water through the chemical formulas for water.

Where Do We Get Our Water?

"Save the Springs"

In the center of the city of 400,000 people is a large park, with a huge, spring-fed public pool. The pool is bordered by the natural rock formations of the creek, but with a concrete wall along one end. Big trees shade the hills along the half-mile stretch of springs. The water is very cool, the city's best offering during the dog days of summer when swimmers come from every part of the city—black, white, Hispanic, Asian, rich, poor, and in between. So in more ways than one, the creek is the heart of the city.

But today, the creek is quiet. A few miles away the park's usual patrons have gathered outside of city hall. They are chanting, "Save Hondo Springs, save Hondo Springs."

The reason for their demonstration is the planned development of land that is part of the creek's watershed. If this area is developed as planned—with a high-tech industry, golf course, and a housing development—environmentalists predict that the creek will receive so much polluted runoff that it will soon be unfit for recreation. Already the creek has had to close on some days following heavy rains because of the high bacterial count. Some others are concerned that the aquifer that serves the entire region does not have a water supply adequate for increased development. The planned development would cover part of the recharge zone for the aquifer. The citizens believe that seepage from the watershed will contribute to contamination of the aquifer. The citizens are pressuring the city council to refuse the developers a permit to further develop the watershed. As the council listens to their speeches, the meeting goes on into the late evening and the wee hours. Not until 4 o'clock the next morning have all of the speakers been heard.

Among those at the hearing is a high school biology teacher, Joanne Li, and two of her students, Leroy Davis and Veronica Garcia. They listen to the hearings thoughtfully and, over the next few weeks, they think about the issues that are raised. There is a lot to think about. Will the city prosper economically without increased development in this area? Is it really so important to have this big swimming area in the middle of town? On the other hand, how can you put a price on the kind of enjoyment that people get in a beautiful natural environment? What about the city's water supply? How is it related to development of the watershed?

The terms used in the scenario above—aquifer and watershed—refer to places where water is found. You can divide the sources of water into two main groups: surface water and ground water. **Surface water** is water that you can see on the Earth's surface: oceans, rivers, lakes, streams, etc. **Ground water** is water found below the Earth's surface.

Surface Water

In the scenario above, the citizens are concerned mainly with surface water, the water in the creek in which they swim. They are aware that water flows into the creek from the surrounding land area above it. The total drainage area where water flows to a common point, such as the creek, is known as a **watershed. Runoff** is water that flows over the watershed after rainfall, snowmelt or irrigation.

Ground Water

The citizens are also concerned with the quality and quantity of ground water in the aquifer in their part of the state. An **aquifer** is a water-bearing layer of rock, gravel or sand below the Earth's surface. Water is taken out of the aquifer by way of pumps and wells; some water returns to the aquifer from the land above it. This land is known as a **recharge zone**. The water seeps through the Earth in the recharge zone to the aquifer below, sometimes taking with it dissolved minerals or metals and other pollutants.

Activity 1-1

- Investigate the sources of water in your community. You will probably need to contact the municipal water authority and you may wish to contact other groups, such as the Environmental Protection Agency or the state water authority. Answer the following questions:
  - What streams and lakes are found in your area?
  - Where is the watershed for these streams and lakes located? How far does it extend from the surface water?
  - From where does the water you use for drinking, washing clothes, bathing, etc. come?
  - Where is the recharge zone for the ground water in your area?
- Evaluate how independent of other communities your community is in its sources of water. Answer the following questions:
  - Does your community use water that is brought in from other areas?
  - Does your community share an aquifer or surface water source with other communities?
  - Do the activities carried out in your community affect the water supply somewhere else? Do the activities carried out elsewhere affect your community's water supply?

The Water Cycle

While doing the preceding activity, you may have realized that water is continually recycled throughout the environment. That's why the use of water in one community is likely to affect neighboring communities in some way. One town's runoff can become part of another town's drinking water.

The continuous circulation of water between the oceans and other surface waters, the atmosphere and the Earth's surface is called the **water cycle** (Figure 1-1). The water cycle is possible because water exists in all of the **three phases of matter**:

- as a **liquid**—in streams, lakes and aquifers
- as a **solid**—in glaciers, frozen surface waters, and the polar ice caps
- as a **vapor**—suspended in the atmosphere.

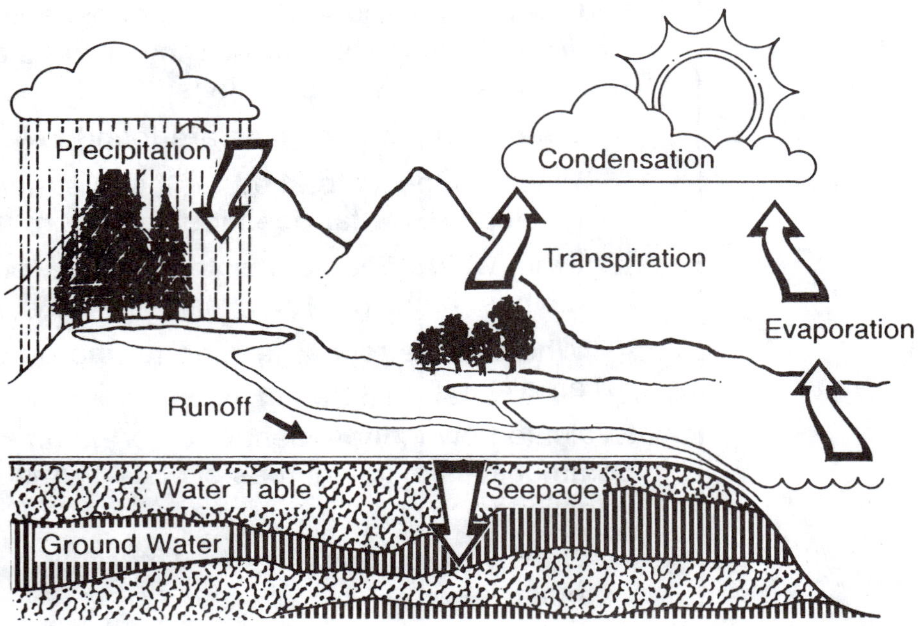

Figure 1-1
The water cycle

How does water move through the environment? Water molecules from surface waters (oceans and land surfaces) evaporate into the air as water vapor. Water vapor enters the atmosphere also by transpiration, which is the loss of water vapor from plant leaves. Water vapor in the atmosphere eventually condenses to produce rain, snow, or other **precipitation**. Rain or other precipitation seeps down to ground water or flows across watersheds into surface water.

Activity 1-2

- Select a creek, stream or pond to study for the duration of this unit. Obtain permission from the owner if the pond is located on private property.
- Fill out Part 1 of the Water Habitat Survey form provided by your teacher and return it to the teacher for approval of your selection.

How Much Water Is Available for Human Use?

Water covers about 75% of the Earth's surface. Some water is found below the Earth's surface. This may seem to be an endless supply of water. However, 97% of all Earth's water is the salt water contained in the oceans. Of the remaining 3% of water, 2% is contained in glaciers and the polar ice caps. The percentage of all of the Earth's water—in ground water and surface water combined—that is available for human consumption is less than 1%.

Throughout history, people have tended to settle and develop cities in areas where fresh water was readily available. In recent decades, population growth and industrialization have increased the demand for fresh water. As a result, access to fresh water is a matter of controversy and struggle in many areas. As water is used and reused for many different purposes by many different people, the quality of water also is affected. As in the scenario at the beginning of this subunit, political battles are fought over who will be allowed to use available water (and the surrounding land that affects the water supply) and for what purpose.

How Do We Use Water?

Activity 1-3

- Conduct an informal poll of adults that you know (parents, neighbors, friends). Find out how water is used in their workplaces. Ask them to be as specific as possible. Also, try to ask people in a variety of occupations.
- As a class, compile the results of your informal poll to come up with a list of ways that water is used. Add to the list any uses that you can think of that take place at school, in the home, or in recreational areas.
- In small groups, examine the class list of water uses and try to group the water uses in some way that makes them easy to understand. In other words, develop categories based on the way that water is used.
- Compare the categories developed by your group with those created by other groups. As a class, decide which system you like the best and why. Keep your list and categories for use in later activities.

  Important Note: Keep in mind that your class poll is not likely to represent a cross section of the entire community. The poll will tell you some uses of water, but may leave out other important uses. Therefore, you may not draw conclusions from this poll about which industries are the biggest water users. If you were trying to evaluate who the major users of water are in your community, you would have to make sure that your sample was representative of all sectors of the town.

Uses of Water in the Vapor Phase

As you've learned by doing the preceding activity, water is used in many different ways. Some uses of water depend upon its being in a vapor phase rather than a liquid phase. Two of these uses are explained briefly below.

One important use of water is based on the pressure it exerts when it is heated to become vapor, also known as steam. When water goes into a vapor phase and is heated to very high temperatures, its molecules move faster. The molecules exert increased pressure on the sides of their container. The pressure of heated steam becomes great enough that it can be used to do work. One of the major uses of steam power is to turn the huge steel turbines of power plants. By its turning, the turbine produces electricity.

Another way that heated steam is used is to heat buildings and homes. Boilers—smaller than the ones used in power plants—heat water to make steam. The steam flows through pipes to radiators that radiate heat to the surrounding air.

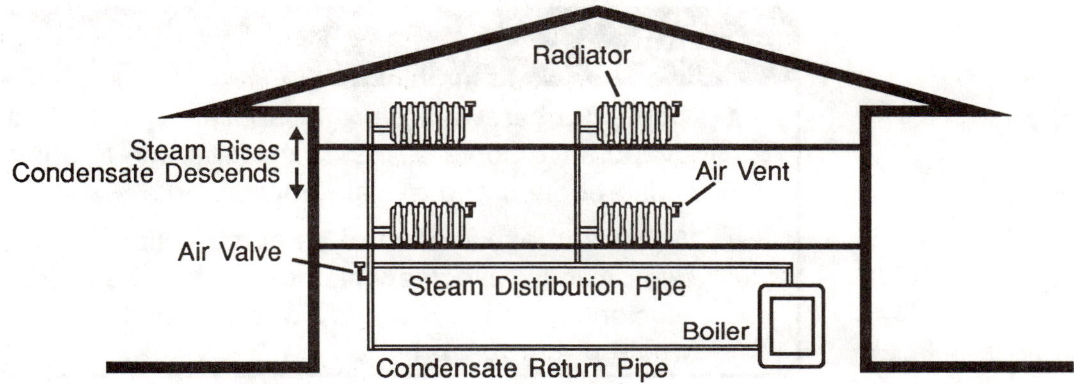

Figure 1-2
Steam heating

Use of Water as a Temperature Regulator and as a Coolant

Water has an important function in living organisms, to cool the body and to regulate its temperature. Vertebrates (animals with backbones) are made up of about two-thirds water. Water cools an animal when it evaporates from a body surface. In many animals, water evaporates either as perspiration or, when the animal pants, as saliva. As water from body surfaces evaporates,the internal temperature of the body tends to drop.

Water absorbs a relatively large amount of heat energy to give a small temperature change. The capability of any substance to absorb heat is an important physical property and is indicated by its heat capacity. **Heat capacity** is the quantity of heat required to change the temperature of one gram of a substance by exactly 1 Celsius degree.

The large heat capacity of water causes temperature changes in an animal's body to occur gradually. For example, during the daytime, as an animal lies in the sun absorbing sunlight, its body temperature slowly increases. Then, after the sun sets, its body temperature slowly decreases.

The way that water functions in living systems also applies to nonliving systems. Water is used to cool through evaporation and conduction. When water evaporates at room temperature, it absorbs energy from the surroundings, making them cooler. You can find out more about how this works through the following activity.

Activity 1-4

- Contact a hardware store or appliance store that sells evaporative coolers. Ask a salesperson to show you one of these coolers and explain how it works.
- Ask for an explanation of an air conditioner. Compare the two devices. Decide which one would be more energy efficient, which one would be more costly, which one you would prefer to own.

Another way that water is used to cool human-made systems is by conduction. **Conduction** is the process in which heat energy flows from an area of higher temperature to an area of lower temperature. Many mechanical or electromechanical systems have materials or parts that must be cooled. Often water is used as a coolant for these systems. One such system is the automobile, in which water is used as a coolant in the radiator. Another system in which water is used as a coolant is in a power-plant condenser. In a condenser, heat moves from steam into cooling water, which then circulates to carry the heat away.

Activity 1-5

- Visit a mechanic and ask about the role of water as a coolant in the automobile. (You will need to make an appointment in advance of your visit.)
- Make a schematic drawing to show how water is used to cool the engine.

JOB PROFILE: POWER PLANT CHEMICAL TECHNICIAN

James C. is a chemical technician for a gas-fired power plant. His main responsibility is water quality. He must ensure that the water supplied to the boiler is ultra-pure. Boiler water has to be pure so that it will not corrode turbine parts or provide resistance to the turbine. James also monitors the quality of cooling water that is used to condense the steam back into water and circulate it back through the system.

Cooling water doesn't have to be as pure as boiler water, but with any water system, impurities can wear parts quickly and clog tubes. Cooling water is pumped through a network of pipes in the condenser. Steam in the condenser passes over the tubes. As the cooling water absorbs heat from the steam, the steam condenses into water on the outside of the tubes. The cooling water flows back into a holding pond until it loses its heat to the air and then is returned to the nearby river.

Much of James' time is spent in sampling, testing and monitoring water quality. James sits in front of a computer in the lab and checks data that is automatically fed from the gauges and machines in the plant. He looks at the data sheets for any reading that is outside of the ordinary. He also makes the rounds of the plant, checking gauges and meters to make sure that they confirm his computer readings. As a third method of checking, James takes water samples at strategic locations throughout the plant and tests them in the laboratory. James has a two-year degree in chemistry technology from a technical institute.

Use of Water to Transport Materials

Because liquid water is fluid (capable of flowing), it can be used to transport substances. On a large scale, boats and barges carry cargo down rivers and in canals. On a smaller scale, water is used to transport materials through pipelines in some industrial settings. Human wastes are carried away from our homes and workplaces to waste treatment plants by means of water. On a still smaller scale—the molecular level—water is used to transport nutrients and wastes to and from cells in animals and plants (Figure 1-3).

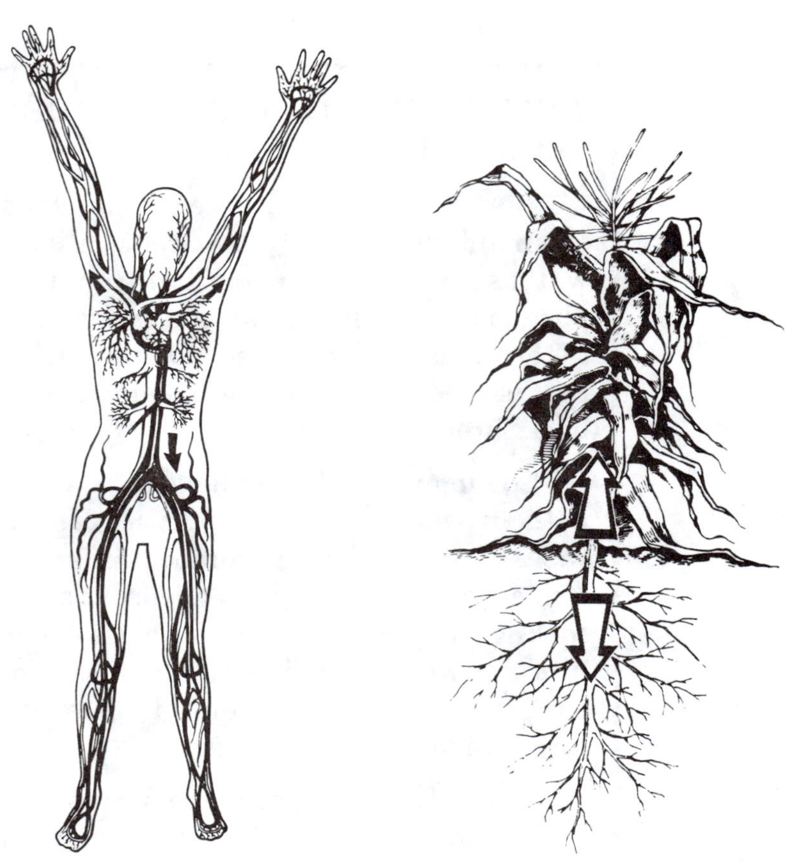

Figure 1-3 Water flow in animals (blood) and plants

Suspensions, Colloidal Suspensions and Solutions

Even though we are talking about all these forms of transport as if they can be easily compared, they differ in some important ways. Some of the substances being carried in water are very large; some are about as small as the water molecules themselves. The behavior of particles in water varies partly according to their size. Three types of mixtures of materials in water are called suspensions, colloidal suspensions and solutions.

In the case of human wastes, the particles of feces that are carried in the water break down into rather small pieces by the time they get to the treatment plant, but they are still bigger than water molecules. Such mixtures—in which the substance in the water is so different in size from that of a water molecule that it has a tendency to settle out—are called **suspensions**. In wastewater treatment plants, wastewater is channeled into settling ponds in which dirt and fecal matter fall to the bottom of the pond, forming a layer of sludge.

Sometimes a substance in water is small enough that it doesn't tend to settle out, but its particles are larger than water molecules. Mixtures like this are called colloidal suspensions. In **colloidal suspensions**, the substance in the water is kept permanently suspended.

Colloidal suspensions are found in nature and in the commercial world. The blood of vertebrate animals is 90% water, which holds proteins and other large molecules in colloidal suspension. Many food products are colloidal suspensions of a liquid in a liquid, called **emulsions**. For example, mayonnaise is an emulsion of vinegar and oil, with egg yolk added to maintain the emulsion.

Activity 1-6

- Divide the class into two groups.
- Using a recipe and materials provided by your teacher, have one group make mayonnaise (using egg yolk) and the other group make salad dressing of vinegar and oil (without egg yolk).
- Refrigerate the mayonnaise and salad dressing for 24 hours.
- Draw a picture of how you think the particles in the mayonnaise and the salad dressing are behaving.
- Answer the following questions:
  - What happens to the vinegar and oil without egg yolk?
  - What seems to be the function of the egg yolk?

Sometimes water carries substances in mixtures called solutions. Often the particles in solutions are about the same size as the water molecules themselves, although they may be larger. In **solutions**, the molecules of the substance that is being dissolved (called the **solute**), are distributed evenly among the molecules of the dissolving medium (called the **solvent**). Solutes may be gaseous, liquid or solid (Figure 1-4).

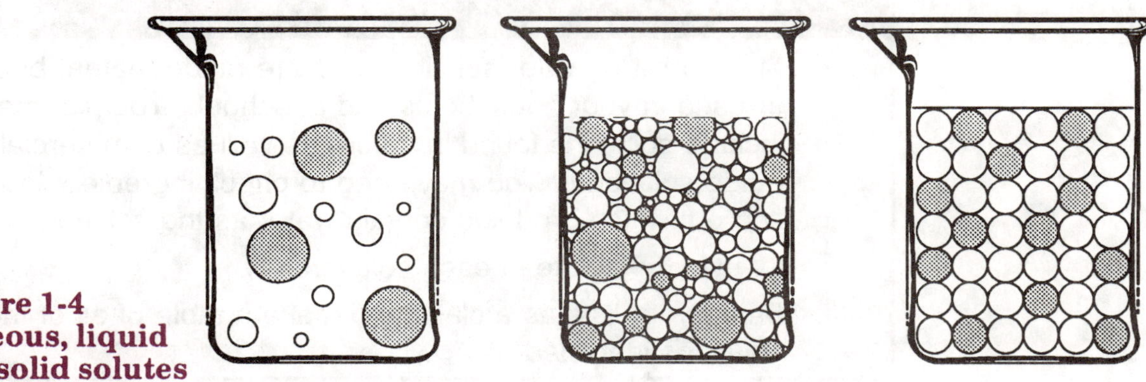

Figure 1-4
Gaseous, liquid and solid solutes

Many nutrients and wastes that are transported in animal bodies are transported in solution. For example, when carbon dioxide is released from cells inside the body, most of it is dissolved into the blood and carried to the lungs where it is released into the air.

JOB PROFILE: PHARMACY TECHNICIAN

Rosa C. is a pharmacy technician. She works in a small pharmacy under the close supervision of a pharmacist.

One part of her job that Rosa likes very much is called compounding. She mixes powders, emulsions and solutions according to instructions given to her by the pharmacist. Compounding requires very specific techniques of mixing and measuring that are standard procedures used in pharmacy. "Sometimes we mix therapeutic skin lotions or we mix powders that are to be taken internally," says Rosa. "Preparing medications is not like baking a cake; you don't just dump everything in and stir. You have to use pharmacy technique."

Rosa learned her job from the pharmacist, and she learned it on the job. She now thinks that it would be interesting to take a chemistry course at the local community college. "I was never interested before," she explains, "but now I'd like to know about different types of chemicals and how they interact."

Suspensions, colloidal suspensions and solutions are different ways in which materials can be distributed and also transported in water. Of these three types of mixtures, solutions are the type that give water its greatest usefulness.

Use of Water as a Solvent

Activity 1-7

- Make a list of water solutions that are made, eaten, bought or used in your households and at school. Your list may include solutions found in nature as well as commercially made solutions. You may need to check ingredient labels to find out which products contain water as the solvent.
- Identify the solute in each solution.
- Share your lists as a class and make a table of all of the solutions identified.

Water's ability to act as a solvent is the basis for many of its uses in nature. We have already mentioned that blood, composed largely of water, is used to transport nutrients and waste products in the body. Water carries minerals from the soil into the cells of plants. Nutrients and carbon dioxide dissolve into the water inside plants, also.

Water is used as a solvent in many commercial products, from food and medicines to household cleaners. Sugar is dissolved into water to make many beverages: lemonade, iced tea and many sodas. Saline is a salt solution used for many medical applications; it is the basic substance into which many medicines are dissolved to be given intravenously (into the vein). Many soaps and detergents dissolve into water (and also attract oil, allowing it to be washed away).

Two important types of solutions are acidic solutions and basic solutions.

Acids and Bases

Acids are substances that, when they are mixed with water, react to form hydronium ions: H_30^+. (You may remember from other units that ions are particles that carry a positive or negative charge. An ion is formed when an atom or a group of atoms gains or loses electrons.)

Many foods contain acids. Oranges and lemons contain citric acid. Souring milk contains lactic acid. Fermented cider forms acetic acid. Many acids are used in industry. One of the most important is sulfuric acid. It is used in petroleum refining, steel processing, and fertilizer production. Phosphoric acid and nitric acid are two other important industrial chemicals; they are used primarily in making fertilizers.

Bases are substances that form hydroxide ions, OH^-, when they are mixed with water. Bases are found in nature and are also commercially prepared. Several basic solutions are found in most people's homes. For example, household ammonia is a basic solution used for cleaning floors and other surfaces. Milk of magnesia is found in many home medicine cabinets and is used as a stomach antacid to treat indigestion.

You will learn more about acids and bases and their interactions in Subunit 4 of this unit.

Use of Water as a Habitat

Water provides a **habitat**, or place to live, for many species of organisms. Most of these live in the oceans, which cover about three-fourths of the Earth's surface. Others inhabit the freshwater lakes, rivers and streams that cover a little over two percent of the Earth's surface.

When most people think of marine life, they think about whales and dolphins, shrimp and snapper, all the fish and sea animals that you can see. But there is another level of marine life—a microscopic level. In the surface waters of the ocean—the first 100 meters or so—live microscopic organisms called **plankton**. Plankton provide food for fish and other larger organisms, and together, plankton and the organisms that eat plankton provide food for even larger organisms, some of which live below the surface waters where sunlight does not penetrate. The plankton are thus the important basis for the **food pyramid** of the ocean (Figure 1-5).

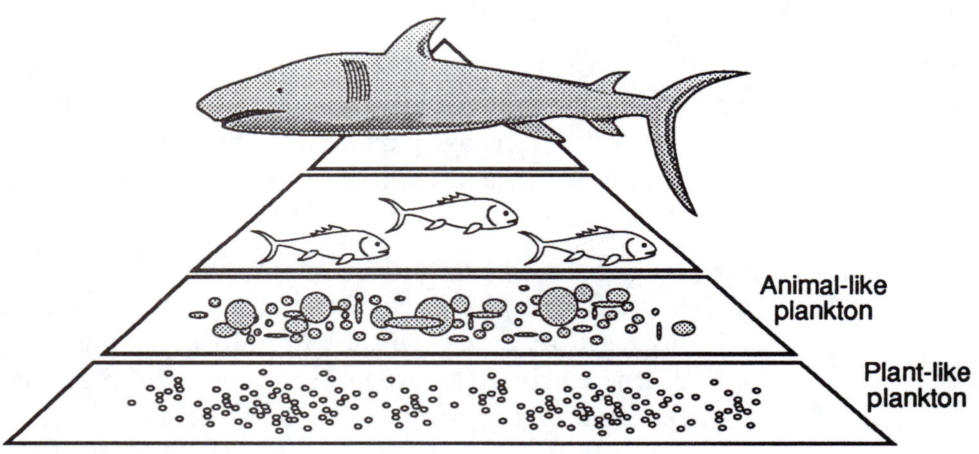

Figure 1-5 Food pyramid of the ocean

Plant-like plankton are responsible for about 40% of all the photosynthesis that takes place on the Earth. Thus they are important users of carbon dioxide and producers of oxygen. Animal-like plankton, feeding on the plant-like plankton, consume oxygen and produce carbon dioxide.

Along the coasts of the continents, the shallow waters of the oceans provide a habitat to large concentrations of aquatic life. These areas are important fisheries and breeding areas for many oceanic species, some of which provide food for human beings. About 5% of the world's food supply now comes from the oceans. Fish are also harvested from freshwater lakes and streams.

Effects of Dispersants on Wildlife

Microscopic plankton that live in ocean waters and provide food to larger marine life were a matter for concern in the debate over how to clean up Prince William Sound after the Exxon Valdez oil spill in 1990.

Two major kinds of control for the spill were undertaken: mechanical control and chemical dispersants. Mechanical control refers to a process of encircling the slick and skimming off the oil; this method was used in Prince William Sound, but the spill was too big for it to do the job alone.

Dispersants also were used to clean up Prince William Sound. Dispersants cause oil to separate and roll up into tiny droplets; in this form it is unable to coat birds and mammals. However, dispersants do stay in the environment, and their long-term effects are not completely understood. Lab and field studies indicate that dispersants are less hazardous than concentrated crude oil. Marine biologists worry that whatever remains in the water—the toxic components of oil and the dispersants—will be absorbed by plankton and have adverse effects and/or work its way up the food chain to affect other marine life.

In recent decades, ocean coastal waters have been threatened by runoff from agricultural, industrial, and other activities. Freshwater bodies of water are less stable than the oceans and have been very vulnerable to human pollution. You will read more about the pollution of water habitats in Subunit 4 of this unit.

An essential factor in the survival of aquatic life is the diffusion of oxygen into water. Oxygen diffuses from the air into water and therefore becomes available to aquatic organisms. The ability of an oceanic area or a freshwater lake to support aquatic life can be measured, in part, by the amount of oxygen dissolved into the water.

The amount of oxygen dissolved in water is called the **dissolved oxygen (dO_2) concentration**. Dissolved oxygen is measured in milligrams per liter of water (mg/l) or parts per million of oxygen to water (ppm). Dissolved oxygen levels vary according to amounts of dissolved or suspended solids in the water, types and numbers of plants, amount of light that penetrates the water, water temperature, motion of the water, and altitude.

Use of Water for Recreation

A day at the lake or the beach seems to be enjoyed by people of all ages. Even though we humans seem poorly adapted to the water—we can't breathe in it, and our skin wrinkles up after less than an hour in it—we still like it (Figure 1-6). Why is this so?

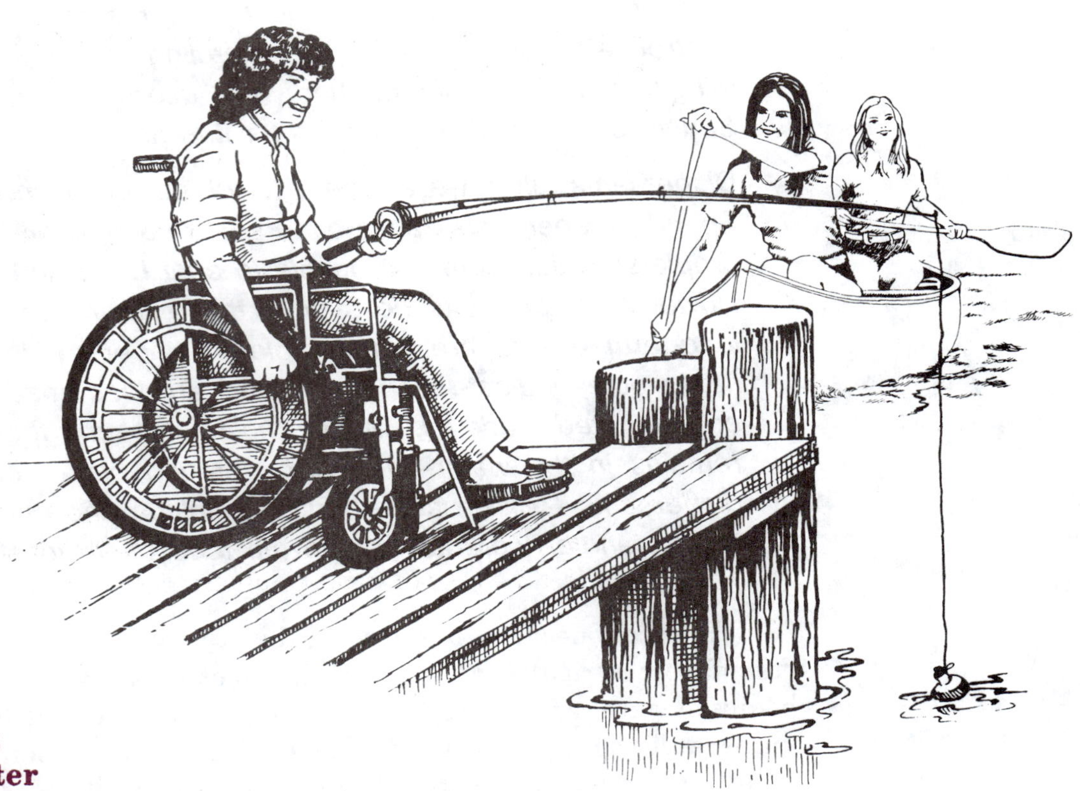

Figure 1-6
Use of water for recreation

One reason we enjoy water may have to do with its density. Density is the mass of a unit volume of material. In other words, density is ratio of mass to volume. It is expressed mathematically as—

$$D = m/v$$ **Equation 1-1**

The density of water is used as a standard by which to compare the density of other materials. The density of water is 1 gram/milliliter. You can compare the density of water to that of other materials if you first find their density using Equation 1.

Activity 1-8

- Find the density of a block of marble measuring 3 cm x 4 cm x 7 cm and weighing 450 grams. Find the volume first by multiplying the dimensions. Then divide the mass by the volume. How much greater is the density of the marble than the density of water?
- Find the density of evaporated milk if 384 cm^3 weighs 411 grams. How does its density compare with that of water?
- Determine the procedures you would use to find the density of the following materials. Compare your procedures with those suggested by others in the class and decide as a class which one might work the best.
  - A bar of soap
  - Whole milk
  - Ice

We are buoyant—that is, we have a tendency to float—in water but not in air because the density of water is greater than the density of air. Do you think that the density of our bodies is closer to that of air or to that of water?

Activity 1-9

- Divide the class into four or five groups.
- In each group, develop a guideline that can be used to predict what materials will float in water and what materials will sink in water. The guideline may be stated in words, shown in a diagram, or expressed as a formula.
- Compare the guidelines developed by each group. Decide on what kind of knowledge or information each guideline is based. Decide which guidelines you think are true and which expressions are clearest.

How Does the Structure of Water Affect the Way It Can Be Used?

After examining all of the uses of water, you may be amazed at how many ways water can be put to work and enjoyed, not to mention the central role it plays in keeping alive plants and animals. Why is water so useful? What is the secret of this unique material that is so essential to life on Earth?

Chemical Formulas for Water

The secret of any material is found in its molecular structure, and water is no exception. The proportion of elements that a molecule contains and the arrangement of the atoms in a molecule give the compound its unique properties. The proportion and arrangement can be expressed in three kinds of chemical formulas—an empirical formula, a molecular formula and a structural formula.

- An **empirical formula** is the simple ratio of the elements in the compound.
- A **molecular formula** gives the number of each type of atom in a molecule of a compound.
- A **structural formula** is the number of atoms of each element and their arrangement in the molecule of a substance.

Empirical Formula

The empirical formula for water is H_2O. It tells us that water has two hydrogen atoms for every one oxygen atom, a ratio of 2 to 1. The empirical formula does not tell how many atoms of each element are in the molecule—the molecular formula does that. It does not tell us how the atoms are bonded together—the structural formula does that.

How do we know the empirical formula for water? Where do these numbers come from? The empirical formula for water, or for any other compound can be calculated if you know the percent composition of each element in the compound. Calculating the empirical formula can be useful if you're trying to find out about an unfamiliar compound.

Activity 1-10

- Use the information and the steps given below to calculate the empirical formula for water.

  Percent composition by weight of water:

  Oxygen = 88.8102%

  Hydrogen = 11.1898%

  Here are the steps involved in calculating the empirical formula:

  1. Convert the percent composition to grams of each element per 100 grams of the compound.
  2. Find the atomic weight of each element using the periodic table.
  3. Divide the grams of each element per 100 grams of the compound by the atomic weight.
  4. Divide the smallest number in the ratio of elements into each of the other numbers to get the smallest possible number ratio.
  5. If the smallest number ratio has any mixed numbers in it, multiply each number in the smallest number ratio by the denominator of the fraction in the mixed number to get the smallest whole number ratio.

Molecular Formula

The molecular formula of a compound gives the number of atoms of each element in a molecule of the compound. You can determine the molecular formula for a compound if you know the empirical formula and the molecular weight of the compound. The molecular weight is the weight in grams of one mole (6.02×10^{23} molecules) of the compound.

Activity 1-11

- Using the information and the steps given below, calculate the molecular formula for water.
  The molecular weight of water is 18.01528 grams per mole.
  Here are the steps involved in calculating the molecular formula:
  1. Determine the empirical formula of the compound (see Activity 1-10).
  2. Calculate the empirical formula weight of the compound by multiplying the atomic weight of each element in the compound times the number of that element in the ratio; then add those products together.
  3. Divide the molecular weight of the compound by the empirical formula weight.
  4. Multiply the factor from #3 times the smallest whole number ratio of the empirical formula.

If you did Activity 1-11, you discovered that the molecular formula for water is the same as the empirical formula—H_2O. This is not the case for all compounds. In Activity 1-12, you determine the empirical and molecular formulas for ethane. For ethane (as for most compounds) these formulas are different.

Activity 1-12

Molecular Formula of Ethane

Ethane is 79.8732% by weight carbon and 20.1268% by weight hydrogen. The gram atomic weight of carbon is 12 grams/mole and the gram atomic weight of hydrogen is 1.00794 grams/mole. The molecular weight of ethane is 30.0476 grams/mole.

- Calculate the molecular formula for ethane.
- Calculate the empirical formula for ethane.

Structural Formula

The structural formula of a compound is the most informative of its chemical formulas. It tells us how the elements in the molecule are arranged. In addition, sometimes information about the angles between bonds and the lengths of bonds is given. The structural formula is not calculated from one or two pieces of data like the empirical and molecular formulas. It is the result of many years of scientific investigation, using many different techniques of observation.

The structural formula for water is shown in Figure 1-7. As you can see, water is made up of one oxygen atom and two hydrogen atoms. Each water molecule is shaped like a triangle with a 105° hydrogen-oxygen-hydrogen bond angle.

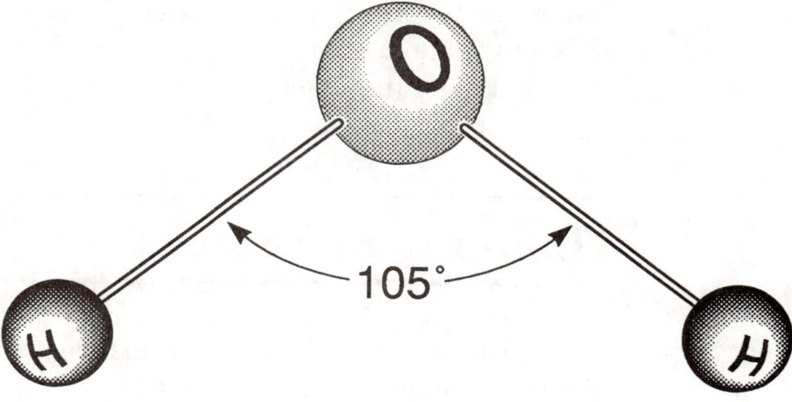

Figure 1-7 Structural formula for water

What is keeping the atoms of hydrogen and the atom of oxygen together in the molecule? To find out, you need to understand more about the chemical bonds of water.

Polarity of Water

You may remember from previous reading that every atom consists of a central nucleus surrounded by electrons. The nucleus contains positively charged particles called protons. The protons attract an equal number of negatively charged particles called electrons. The electrons are found at various distances outside the nucleus.

When atoms bond together, they may share electrons, or they may transfer electrons from one atom to another. In the case of water, the electrons are shared. Each hydrogen atom shares an electron with oxygen.

The shared electrons of a water molecule do not lie exactly between the oxygen nucleus and the nucleus of each hydrogen atom. Instead, they cluster a little closer to the oxygen nucleus. As a result, the oxygen atom is a little bit negatively charged, and the hydrogen atoms are a little bit positively charged. Therefore water is polar. It acts somewhat like a very tiny magnet.

When water falls to the ground from the sky, it acts like a magnet to particles which can dissolve into it. Air and dust move into the drops of water as it plummets from the sky. When the drops hit the surface of the ground, they divide into many smaller pieces, increasing their surface area and allowing smaller particles, solids, to become mixed among the water molecules.

The polarity of water is what causes it to attract particles and hold them in solution. Keep in mind that this process does not involve water's breaking down into its two elements and joining with other elements to form new substances. That would be a chemical change. Water is able to hold substances in solution by its polar charges, without changing itself chemically.

Looking Back

About 75% of the Earth's surface is covered with water, most of it in the oceans. However, the greatest source of fresh water is found beneath the Earth's surface in the ground water of aquifers.

Water moves through the environment continuously in what is known as the water cycle. Water enters the atmosphere by evaporation from surface waters and by transpiration of plants. Water vapor in the atmosphere eventually condenses to produce rain, snow, or other precipitation, which falls to the Earth, seeps down to ground water or flows across watersheds into surface water. Thus our water supply is a shared resource.

Water has many useful properties. In its vapor phase, it can be used to heat buildings or made to do work. Because of its high heat capacity, water makes an excellent temperature regulator inside the bodies of animals as well as in industrial systems. Also, water is used for transport inside plant and animal bodies and in industrial systems. Water provides a habitat for thousands of aquatic species, from plankton to great whales.

One of water's most useful properties is its ability to act as a solvent. Water can dissolve other materials well because of the polarity of its molecular structure. The shared electrons of the water molecule cluster a little closer to the oxygen nucleus than to the nuclei of the two hydrogen atoms. As a result, the oxygen atom is a little bit negatively charged, and the hydrogen atoms are a little bit positively charged. Thus water molecules act like tiny magnets to many other particles.

Further Discussion

- Your county is experiencing a severe drought and your local water supply is drying up. You must ration the remaining water supply. Which water uses will you prohibit? Which water uses will you allow? How will you prioritize those uses? What restrictions or limits will you put on the remaining usages? Justify your decisions.
- Most of the water on Earth is salt water from oceans. Many of the dry countries (in the Middle East for example) use desalination (removal of salt) plants to provide fresh water. Discuss the advantages of this compared to other ways of getting fresh water. Are there any disadvantages to this method? Why don't we use desalination plants to supply water for our coastal cities?

Activities by Occupational Area

General

Water Cartography

- Using information obtained from various sources—the local water protection agency, environmental agencies or groups, recreation agencies, etc.—make a simplified map of the surface waters and ground waters in your region, one that can be used to educate students.

Agriculture and Agribusiness

Drought-Resistant Plants/Water-Loving Plants

- Consult with your local agricultural extension agent or an informed plant nursery owner or manager to find out what landscaping plants used in your area are known for their low water use and what plants are known for their high water use.
- Identify and get approval for five or more test plot areas on the school campus. Assign each test plot to a different group in the class. Subdivide each test plot area into two parts. In one part plant high-water-use plants and in the other, plant low-water-use plants.

- Keep a log of the progress of the two types of plants in each test plot over the next several weeks. Note soil types, patterns of rainfall and other precipitation, patterns of runoff, erosion and/or flooding, and growth progress.
- As a class, look at the data log and decide if you can draw any conclusions from it concerning the following: 1) whether the plants performed as predicted, 2) which areas of the campus are more conducive for growing each type of plant, and 3) what growth factors require further investigation.

Agricultural Runoff

- Contact the local office of the Environmental Protection Agency to find out what types of runoff pollution are associated with agricultural activities in your region.
- Contact the local office of the Farm Bureau to find out what types of runoff pollution are associated with agricultural activities in your region.
- As a class, compare the information obtained from each organization. How does it differ? Why do you think it is different? How does each organization support its conclusions? How could you verify the information you were provided?

Health Occupations

Hospital Pharmacy

- Visit a hospital pharmacist and find out what kinds of sterile water solutions are prepared and/or distributed in the hospital. Answer these questions: If the solutions are prepared by the pharmacy, what are the main ingredients? Who prepares the solutions? What kind of precautions are required in preparing such solutions? What kind of chemistry is required?

Temperature Regulation

- Interview a neonatal-care nurse to find out how temperature regulation in premature infants differs from that of adults and from infants carried to term.
- Find out what measures are taken to control the body temperatures of neonates.

Home Economics

Food-Emulsifying Agents

- Visit the local supermarket and identify as many food products as possible in which emulsifying agents are used. (If you have trouble figuring out which additives are emulsifying agents, contact your local home economics extension agent or do some library research on food emulsifiers.)
- Verify the items on each person's list. Give a food prize to the person in your class who comes up with the longest list.

Home Water-Filtering Devices

- Investigate the home water-purification market in your area. Find out what water-filtering devices and water-purification products (such as tablets) are sold.
- Compare the way in which each solution works and decide the advantages and disadvantages of each for solving different kinds of water problems.

Industrial Technology

Cooling Water for Nuclear Power Plants

- Investigate the use of water for cooling in nuclear power plants. You may use the library, or contact a nearby nuclear power plant or write to the U.S. Nuclear Regulatory Commission.
- Answer the following questions and report your findings to the class: How is water used in water-cooled reactors? Is the water contaminated by radiation? Why? What happens to the water while the plant is in operation and after the plant is decommissioned?

Testing for Water Quality

- Contact the Environmental Protection Agency, a local civil engineering firm, regional water-quality board or agency, or other organization that hires environmental technicians to test water quality.
- Interview the person who carries out such tests. Find out what tests are used and what aspect of water quality they indicate.

SUBUNIT 2

How Does Water Support Life?

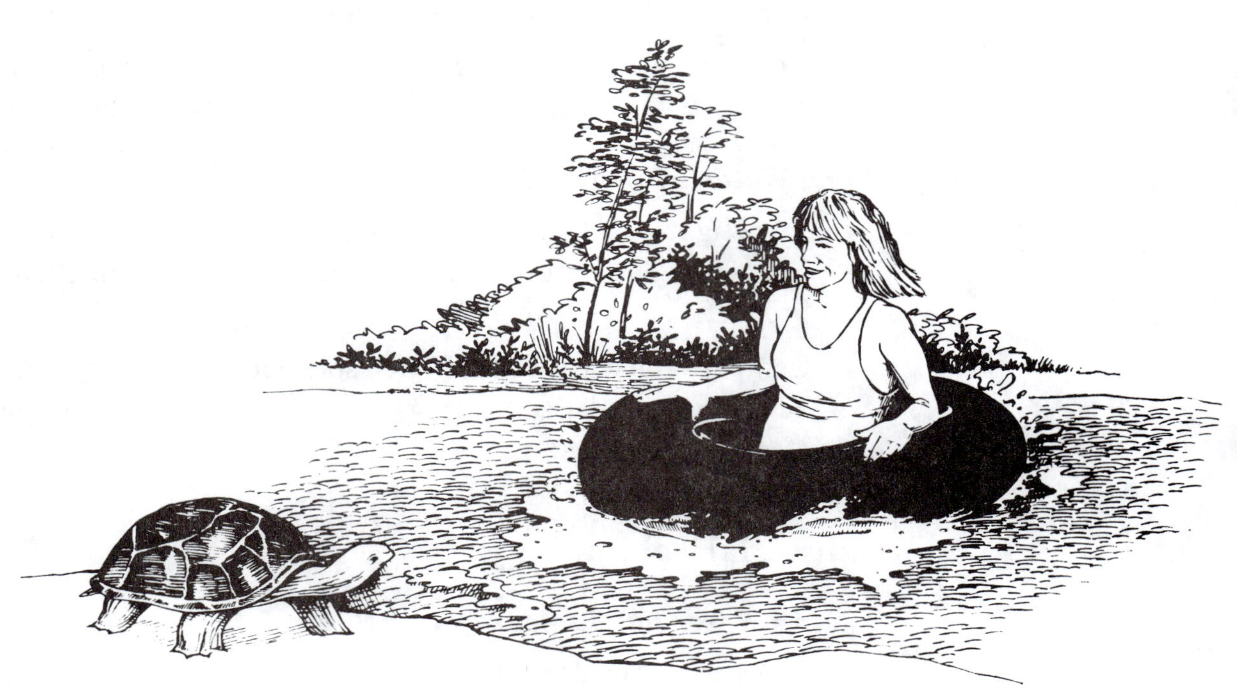

THINK ABOUT IT

- How does the girl in the picture above depend on water to stay alive? How does the turtle depend on water to stay alive?
- What role does water play in maintaining a livable temperature for the girl and the turtle?
- What other functions does water have for these two organisms? How does water support the plants growing by the riverbank?

SUBUNIT OBJECTIVES

After you complete this subunit, you will be able to —

1. **Predict how selected organisms will react to environmental temperature changes, based on the role of water as a temperature regulator.**
2. **Link the physical and chemical properties of water to its function as a transporter of nutrients inside plants and animals.**
3. **Describe the role of water in biochemical reactions in organisms.**
4. **Choose an organism and evaluate its ability to maintain water balance in an extreme condition.**
5. **Recommend strategies for supplying water to livestock.**
6. **Describe how diffusion and osmosis help animals and plants to obtain nutrients and maintain water balance.**

How Does Water Support Life?—An Overview

Hondo Springs (Part 2)

Following the long demonstration and heated hearings at City Hall, the controversy over Hondo Springs continues over several months. During that time, the pool has to be closed numerous times after the early and midsummer rains. The rain brings runoff from housing and commercial developments in the watershed above the springs. City park officials are obliged to close the pool when the fecal coliform count exceeds an acceptable level. Fecal coliform is a count of bacterial life forms that reside in human and animal wastes.

In a first round of hearings during the summer, it seemed that some of the city council members were uneducated about water-quality issues. They knew what the fecal coliform count was, but they seemed unaware of how vital water is to many life forms.

Joanne and her students decide that the council members need more information. They decide to educate the council during the next round of hearings. They begin by doing some library research on water, going through textbooks and articles, reading about water in the leaves of plants, water in cells, and water and kidney function. Then they focus on the springs. They do a survey of life forms in and around the springs: plants, fish, land animals, and microscopic life.

Activity 2-1

- Using the Water Habitat Survey Form provided by your teacher, visit your selected site (approved earlier).
- Fill out Part II "Survey of Life Forms."
- Compare your findings with other class members to see how they are alike and different.

As land animals, we humans sometimes forget that we are two-thirds water. We can't see all of the ways that water keeps us alive. In this subunit, you will explore the different ways that water functions in living systems: as a temperature regulator, a transporter of nutrients, a solvent, and a biochemical reactant and product. You will also find out about how organisms—whether on land or sea or freshwater springs—maintain a relatively constant internal amount of water. This is referred to as maintaining water balance.

What Is the Role of Water in Regulating Temperatures?

Most animal life processes such as oxidation of carbohydrates and protein synthesis can take place only within a narrow temperature range. A change in temperature of only a few degrees can disrupt these processes. Water plays a key role in maintaining body temperature at the desired range.

A Battle Against Fever

On the recommendation of his pediatrician, five-year-old Robbie was just admitted to the hospital for intensive treatment of strep throat. Robbie has had chronic strep throat during the last three months. Each time he has a bout with the strep infection, he is treated with antibiotics and appears to recover, only to become ill again in a few weeks.

Robbie's mother says that he has eaten very little in the last day and a half and has had diarrhea all day. During the last hour, his fever has suddenly risen to 103.5 degrees F.

In the hospital, Robbie's pediatric nurse, Carl, has received orders from his doctor by phone. Carl puts Robbie on intravenous fluids to fight his dehydration and starts him on antibiotics (also given intravenously) to fight his infection. When the nurse's aide, Valerie, comes into Robbie's room, Carl explains what is going on.

"His fever is his body's attempt to kill off his strep infection," says Carl. "But a sudden rise like that can cause a seizure, so we need to get it down as quickly as possible."

"What do we do?" asks Valerie.

"Well, he's too dehydrated from his diarrhea to sweat and cool himself down. We've got him on IV fluids to remedy the dehydration, but in the meantime, we need to remove his clothes and put some cool packs under his arms and at the top of his thighs where the blood flow is high. And we'll need a fan in here to carry away some of the heat. But we have to keep a close eye on him so that he doesn't get chilled. If he starts shivering, his muscles will have to work, and he'll be generating heat all over again."

Carl and Valerie place ice packs on Robbie's body, talking to him all the while to lessen his fear of the hospital and of being sick.

How do we humans and other animals manage to keep our body temperatures stable? The preceding scenario suggests two mechanisms by which the body regulates its own temperature: sweating and shivering. How do these work and in what other ways does the body maintain its proper temperature? How are animals able to live in areas of climate extremes such as deserts or mountaintops? How are we able to withstand seasonal changes from 40°C (104°F) summer days to –20°C (– 4°F) winter weather?

We are able to maintain our body temperatures within a fairly narrow range largely because we have a high water content in our bodies. Water makes up about two-thirds of the bodies of most vertebrates and is an important component of every organism on Earth.

Water's High Heat Capacity

The capability of any substance to absorb heat is an important physical property and is indicated by its heat capacity. Heat capacity involves three quantities:

- heat energy (absorbed or released)
- mass of material that is absorbing or releasing heat energy
- temperature change

When heat energy is applied, a substance with a high heat capacity will have a gradual increase in temperature, and a substance with a low heat capacity will have a quick increase in temperature (see Figure 2-1).

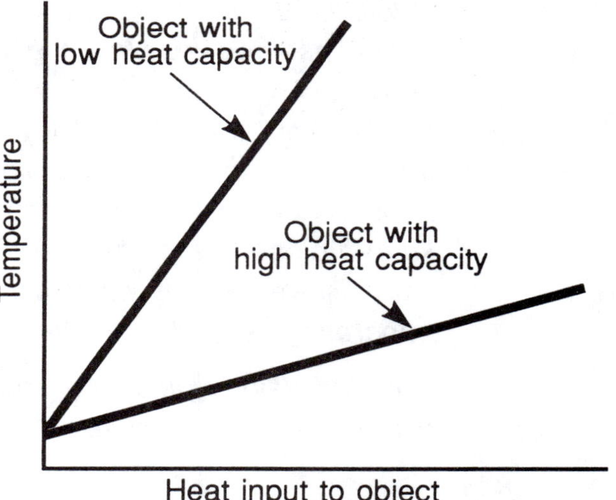

Figure 2-1 Comparison of rate of temperature increase in substances with high and low heat capacities

Heat capacity is defined as the quantity of heat required to change one gram of a substance by exactly one Celsius degree. The units used to measure heat capacity can vary. The energy can be measured in calories or Btu. The mass of an object or quantity of liquid can be expressed in grams or pounds. The temperature change can be expressed in Celsius or Fahrenheit degrees.

You learned in Subunit 1 that the large heat capacity of water causes temperature changes in an animal's body to occur gradually. For example, if a lizard lies in the sun absorbing sunlight, its internal body temperature slowly increases. If the lizard moves behind a rock, its internal body temperature slowly decreases. The water in its body gives up or gains heat slowly. The rate of heat loss or gain depends on the difference between the surrounding air temperature and the body temperature. Because of the high heat capacity of water, a large quantity of heat can be lost or gained for a mere 1° temperature decrease or increase.

Activity 2-2

- Investigate how some organisms respond to environmental temperature changes either by mechanisms regulating their own internal temperature or by other adaptations that allow them to survive temperature extremes.
  - camel
  - pupfish
  - penguin
  - gecko
  - goldfish
  - polar bear
  - javelina
  - yak
  - piranha
  - sparrow
  - oppossum
  - squid
  - llama
  - bat
  - alligator
  - koala bear
  - cockroach
  - bacteria (choose species)

- Share your information with the class. As a class, try to come up with a classification of organisms based on the way internal body temperatures fluctuate or are regulated under changing environmental conditions.

Water's Heat of Vaporization

Besides its ability to store heat and release it slowly, water provides another mechanism for regulating the temperature of many organisms: a high heat of vaporization. Many mammals lower their body temperatures through evaporation by sweating or panting (Figure 2-2) and directly make use of this property of water.

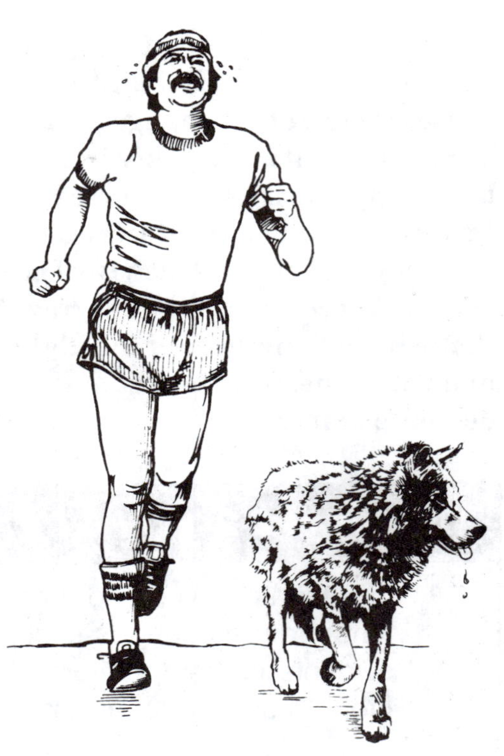

Figure 2-2 Two means of preventing overheating

The heat of vaporization is the heat required to change one gram of liquid water into water vapor. The heat of vaporization of water is fairly high—540 calories per gram. So the evaporation of water through sweating or panting carries quite a bit of heat away from the body.

But what causes us to sweat or a dog to pant when body temperature starts to rise? The answer is that the body has its own thermostat. Just as the air conditioning in a central air system turns on when the indoor air reaches a preset temperature, the body "turns on" certain responses when its internal temperature reaches a certain point.

The body's thermostat is located in the hypothalamus, a part of the brain that, among other functions, senses the temperature of the blood. Normally the human hypothalamus recognizes a preset temperature of 98.6°F.

In the preceding scenario, Robbie's biological thermostat was reset to a higher temperature in response to his bacterial infection. (The reasons for such a fever are not completely understood, but it seems to be the body's attempt to weaken infecting bacteria.) Robbie's normal cooling mechanisms were thus suppressed. His nurse knew fluids and ice packs were needed to lower his temperature. But the nurse was also aware that if Robbie's body temperature went too far below the new preset temperature, his hypothalamus would direct his muscles to increase their activity. The resulting shivering would raise his temperature again.

Water and Temperature Regulation in Plants

Since plants are typically made up of 80% to 90% water, they benefit (as animals do) from the high heat capacity and high heat of vaporization of water. But unlike many vertebrate animals, plants are temperature conformers; their temperature fluctuates with the surrounding temperature. (Fortunately, plant processes such as photosynthesis can take place under much greater extremes of temperature than can many animal life processes.)

For plants, water stress is a much greater threat to survival than is a simple increase in body temperature. The water balance of a plant is, however, ultimately linked to environmental temperature. The higher the air temperature, the greater the evaporation of water from plant tissues. This water loss by evaporation is referred to as transpiration. Many plants retard water loss by structural features such as waxy leaf surfaces and leaf hairs that collect evaporating water droplets to form a water vapor barrier. The water vapor barrier slows down evaporation from within the plant.

In intense heat plants can lose a great deal of water by transpiration, especially through their stomata. If this water loss were not immediately replaced by water from the soil, the plant would wilt (Figure 2-3a) and eventually die. How can plants guard against this? They can do it by closing the stomata of the leaves. With these millions of tiny pores closed, a plant under heat stress can conserve water. But there is a drawback to keeping the stomata closed for too long -- there is no way for carbon dioxide to enter the plant, and so photosynthesis shuts down.

Water may become unavailable to plants even in cold weather. If temperatures are cold enough to freeze soil moisture into ice crystals, plant roots cannot function. As winter approaches, plants of some species drop their leaves. They give up on photosynthesis for the winter, form buds and become dormant (Figure 2-3b).

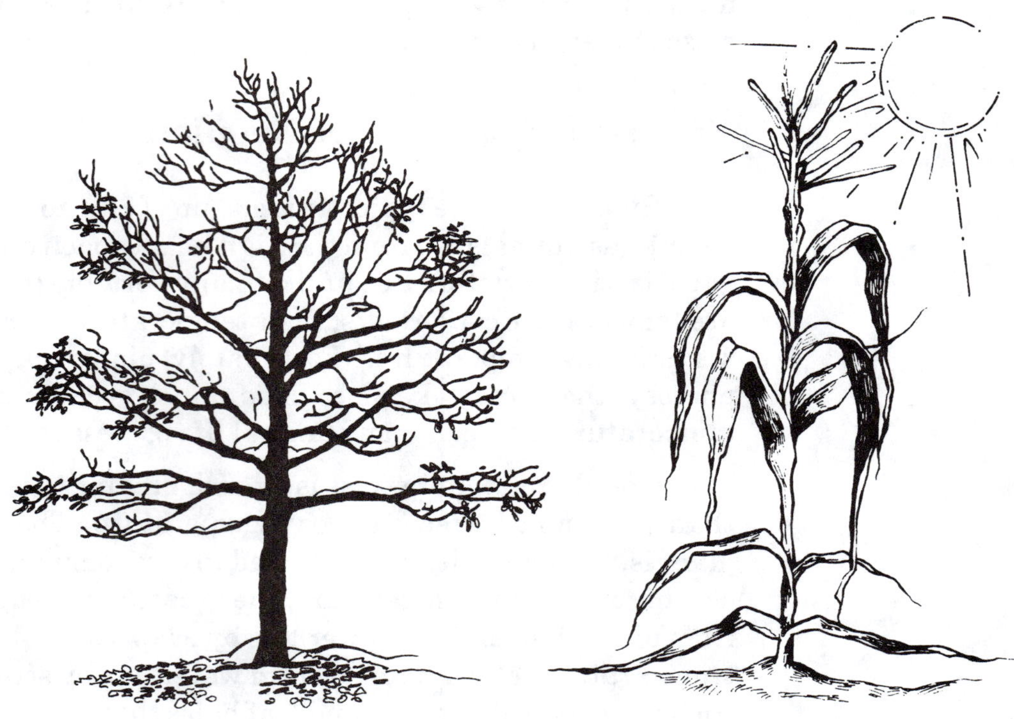

Figure 2-3
Two responses of plants to temperature extremes

What Is the Role of Water in Transporting Nutrients and Other Materials?

Most single-celled organisms have an advantage when it comes to getting the materials needed for life and getting rid of wastes. Their cells obtain nutrients directly from the water environment in which they live and they eliminate wastes directly to that same environment.

For multicellular organisms, it's more complicated to move materials into and out of all the organisms' cells. All cells do not have direct access to the environment. Therefore multicellular organisms must transport water and nutrients to every cell and waste materials from every cell. In plants, water is drawn from soil into the roots, up through the plants' networks of water-transport tubules and out to the leaves. In vertebrates, nutrients and other materials are delivered to cells by way of the fluid highways of the circulatory system. (Blood contains a high proportion of water.)

The term bulk flow is often used to refer to the movement of water (or fluids composed primarily of water) in a mass within plants and animals. The movement of blood in the circulatory system and the movement of water through the stems of plants are both examples of bulk flow.

What Behaviors of Water Are at Work in Living Systems?

For all organisms—one-celled amoebas, or multicellular worms, clams, insects vertebrate animals and plants—water is the medium by which needed materials are carried. So in explaining exactly how materials are transported in living things, you have to be aware of the properties of water and water solutions. In other words, water behaves in the same way whether it is in nonliving systems or in living systems. Several behaviors of water are important in the movement of materials in the body; chief among them are diffusion and osmosis.

Diffusion

Diffusion is the process by which particles (molecules, ions, or atoms) of a substance spread out to occupy a space uniformly. You can observe diffusion by doing the following activity.

Activity 2-3

- Fill a laboratory sink with water. Dump into the sink a small amount of dye provided by your teacher.
- Observe the dye in the water. What happens to it? Why do you think that it behaves the way that it does?

Diffusion is a movement of particles from an area of higher concentration to an area of lower concentration. Concentration refers to the number of molecules or atoms of a substance relative to the space that the substance occupies. In the case of solutions, concentration refers to the amount of solute in a solution. A solution with a lot of solute is said to be highly concentrated. A solution with a small amount of solute is said to be less highly concentrated, or more diluted.

Diffusion is caused by the random motion of the particles that make up the substance. As the particles move randomly, some of them move toward the center of concentration (Figure 2-4a).

However, as particles move closer to the center, they collide with more and more molecules. The collisions divert the molecules away from the center of concentration and toward the less concentrated areas of the available volume (Figure 2-4b). This process continues until the available volume has an even distribution of particles of the substance (Figure 2-4c).

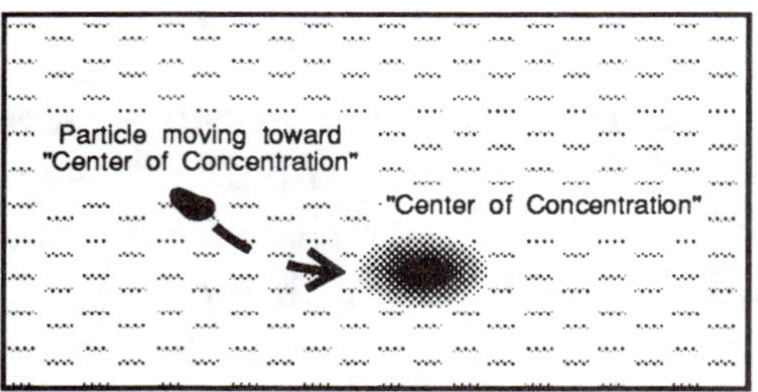

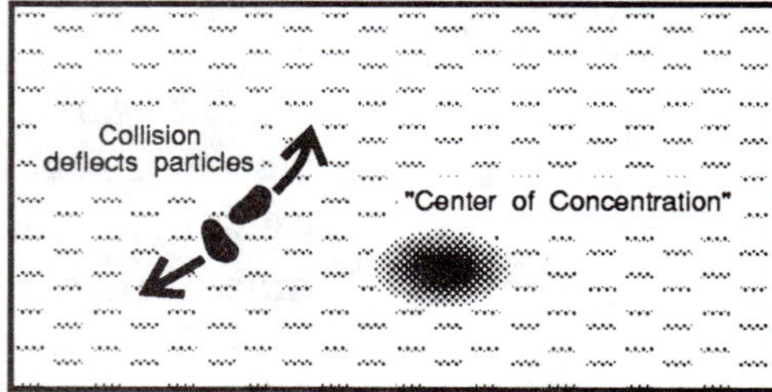

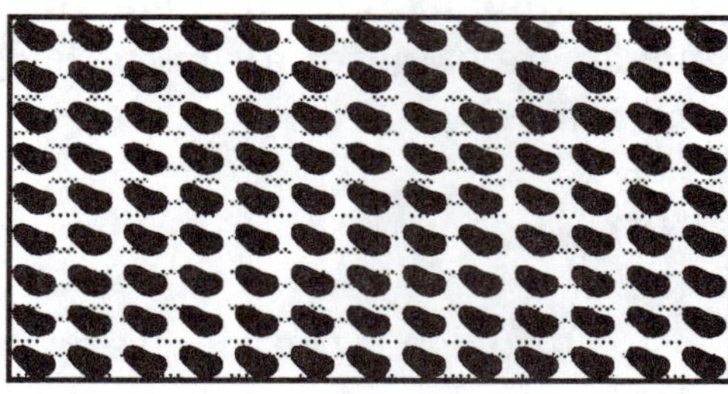

Figure 2-4 Stages in the process of diffusion

You have seen that particles will diffuse from an area of greater concentration into an area of lesser concentration. What happens to this tendency to diffuse when molecules or atoms confront a membrane? The short answer to this question is, it depends on the molecule and the type of membrane. You can find out what happens with one type of membrane in the following activity.

Activity 2-4

- Stretch a piece of dialysis membrane given to you by your teacher across the wide part of a glass funnel to make a container. Slowly pour the container about 1/4 full with a salt solution (3%).
- Immerse the container of salt solution into a beaker of distilled water. Observe what happens and discuss as a class what you think are the reasons for it.

The dialysis membrane used for the preceding activity is permeable to both water and the solute, salt. Therefore the diffusion process continues across the membrane until the diffusing particles are evenly distributed on both sides of the membrane.

JOB PROFILE: HEMODIALYSIS TECHNICIAN

Irene C. is a hemodialysis technician in a clinic that treats 400 patients for chronic kidney failure per week. Irene is responsible for 4-6 patients at a time.

"The dialyzer is like an artificial kidney," explains Irene. "The dialyzer is a semipermeable membrane encased in a clear tube about 8 inches long and 2 to 3 inches wide. The membrane is composed of tiny tubular fibers. The patient's blood comes into the fibers (something like the way blood flows into capillaries). The dialysate is a saline solution that flows into the dialyzer and surrounds the fibers. The two fluids, the blood and dialysate, flow across each other in the dialyzer but they do not mix."

Irene has a high school diploma and has been through the clinic's six-week training course for dialysis technicians. She understands how the process works and explains it to us. "Dialysis is a process of diffusion. Solvents go from areas of high concentration to areas of lower concentration. Dialysate has a low concentration of electrolytes. The patient's blood contains waste products with a high concentration of electrolytes. The waste products of the blood are drawn off through the semipermeable membrane into the dialysate. That's how the blood gets cleaned of waste products."

"My job is to receive the patients, hook them up to the dialysis machine, monitor their status during the 4-or 5-hour-long dialysis process, and disconnect them from the machine when they are finished," says Irene.

Receiving them means weighing them and checking but not taking their temperature and blood pressure," she goes on. "A nurse puts the catheter into their arm. Then I connect the dialyzer and blood-flow lines to the machine. I record the patient's temperature, pulse rate and blood pressure every 30 minutes, and I also observe and record their general condition. I check the machine, too—the pressure gauges, flow meters, and other indicators."

Irene reflects on the job. "It's a job that requires that you stay on your toes. With 4 to 6 patients to watch all the time, you don't have a chance to let your attention wander. At the same time, you have to remember to be kind to the patients. This isn't an enjoyable process for them, especially if you treat them like part of the machinery. I try to make them comfortable and to respect their feelings."

Osmosis

In the cells of organisms, the diffusion of water across cell membranes can create problems for cells. Cell membranes are different from the dialysis membrane used in Activity 2-4 in an important way: Water can diffuse across most cell membranes, but same solutes cannot. Cell membranes are thus said to be selectively permeable. Selectively permeable membranes allow some molecules to pass through and keep others out.

Osmosis is the diffusion of water across a selectively permeable membrane, from an area of greater water concentration to an area of lesser water concentration. You can observe the process of osmosis in the following activity.

Activity 2-5

- Stretch a piece of dialysis membrane given to you by your teacher across the wide part of a glass funnel to make a container. Slowly pour the container about 1/4 full, this time with a starch solution (3%).
- Immerse the container of starch solution into a beaker of distilled water. Observe what happens and discuss as a class what you think are the reasons for it.

In the preceding activity, the membrane allows water molecules to pass through it, but it keeps out the starch molecules. Water molecules strike both sides of the membrane. On the solution side of the membrane, starch molecules also strike the membrane. The side with pure water is hit with more water molecules than the solution side (because all of the molecules on the pure-water side are water molecules but only some of the molecules on the solution side are water molecules). Because more water molecules are striking the membrane on the water side, more water molecules pass through the membrane from the water side to the solution side.

As the process of osmosis continues, the concentration of the starch solution decreases because more water passes into the solution. However, if starch cannot pass through the membrane, the concentrations on the two sides of the membrane cannot become equal. What then causes osmosis to stop?

Osmosis continues until the pressure on the solution side of the membrane is high enough to stop the process. As more water molecules pass into the solution, there is a corresponding increase in the number of times per second that water molecules strike the membrane. This increase causes more water molecules to pass back from the solution side to the pure-water side of the membrane. At the point of equilibrium, the rate at which molecules are passing from the solution side to the pure-water side is equal to the rate at which molecules are passing from the pure-water side to the solution side.

What creates the pressure on the solution side of the membrane? Pressure can build up in two different ways, depending upon whether the system is closed or open (Figure 2-5).

If a solution is completely enclosed in a membrane, pressure builds up inside the membrane as more and more water enters the solution (Figure 2-5a). If the membrane is not able to withstand the pressure, it will rupture before equilibrium is reached.

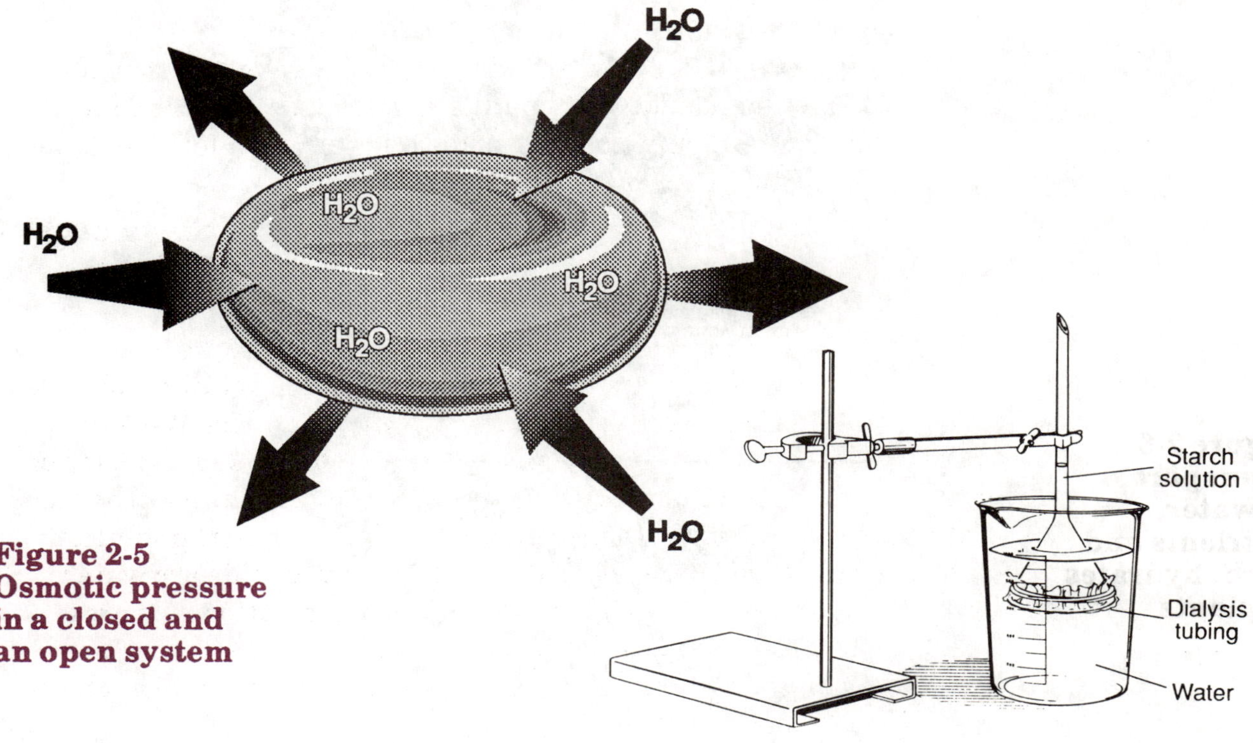

Figure 2-5 Osmotic pressure in a closed and an open system

What creates pressure in an open system? In an open system such as the one in Activity 2-5, the level of the solution will rise as water crosses the membrane into the solution (Figure 2-5b). In such a system, which is similar to that found in plants, pressure is created by the density of fluid, the gravity acting on the fluid, and the height of the fluid. As the level of the solution increases, the pressure also increases. When the height of the solution is sufficient to cause the pressure necessary for equilibrium, the osmotic pressure of the solution has been reached.

How Does Water Carry Materials to the Cells of Plants?

In plants, water carries nutrients from the soil into the plant through the roots, up the stem or trunk and out to the leaves. Water also transports carbohydrates (manufactured during photosynthesis) from the leaves and down through the stem into the roots (Figure 2-6).

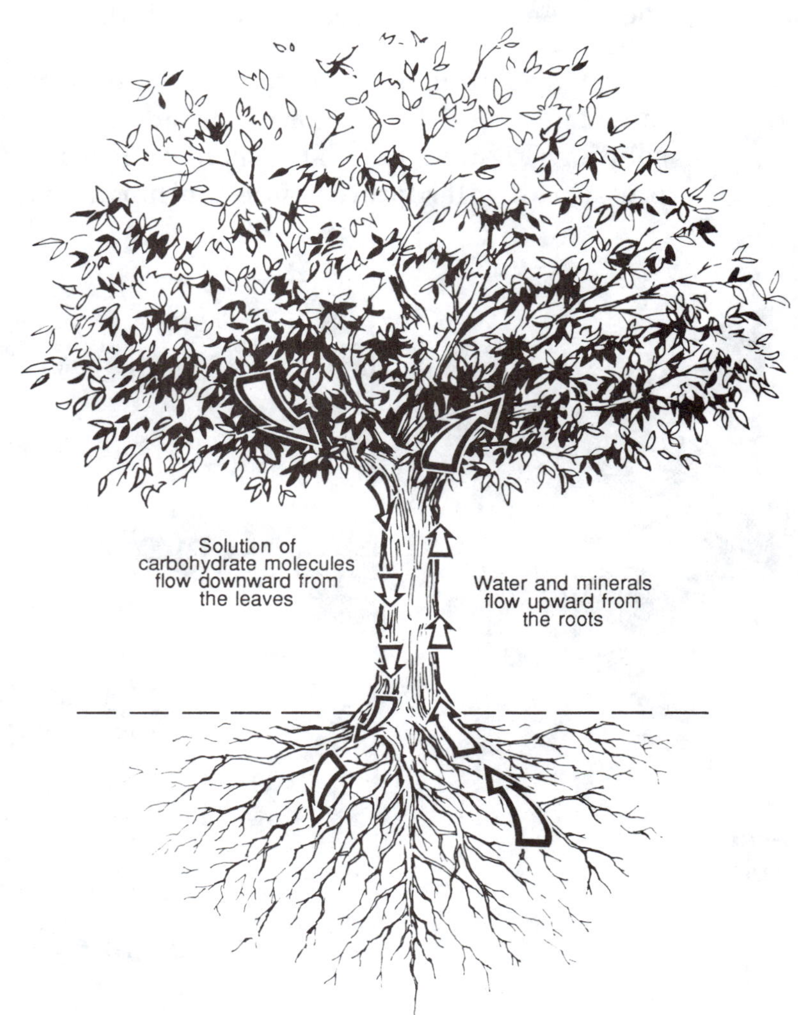

Figure 2-6 Transport of water, nutrients and carbohydrates in plants

JOB PROFILE: COTTON FARMERS IN WEST TEXAS

Jack and Naomi W. are cotton farmers in the relatively dry region of Midland, Texas. Together with their son, who farms the adjacent acreage and is gradually assuming more and more of the total farm, they have about 1500 acres of land. Jack and Naomi are almost seventy years old, but they still experiment and learn new things about farming. Every year they run test plots. They experiment with new seed strains, irrigation and planting methods, insect control, or any other factor that might lead to more cotton per acre at a lower cost.

One change that Jack and Naomi have made in recent years is from sprinkle to drip irrigation systems. Jack explains that a few years ago, he ran test plots to find out which method was more effective. "Common sense told me that we were losing a lot of water to evaporation in sprinkle irrigation," he explains. "But the test plots showed me that drip irrigation could increase my yields to give a 50% profit increase, even after subtracting the cost of pumps, piping and valves!"

Naomi continues, "Getting water to our crops is a major part of our costs here in West Texas. Increasing the efficiency of our water use meant an increase in profits."

As stated earlier, water movement in a plant is largely a process of bulk flow. The plant is like a tube through which water flows. However, you may wonder how a plant—especially a tall tree—is able to pull water up to its leaves against the force of gravity. Water rises in the plant primarily as a result of two kinds of pressure: suction pressure and root pressure.

- A negative pressure, or suction pressure, is created when water evaporates from the leaves of the plant during transpiration; this negative pressure pulls up on the water columns in the stem and roots. This pressure is sometimes called transpiration pull.
- Pressure is created by the difference in the concentration of solutes inside the root cells compared with the concentration of solutes in the soil. Water moves by osmosis into the area in which solutes are more concentrated; that is, into the roots. This pressure is sometimes called root pressure. Root pressure can bring so much water into the plant that water and minerals are forced out along the margins of the leaves.

Activity 2-6

- Grow or obtain two small bean plants; put each one in a separate container. Label them A and B.
- For a period of several days, water plant A with distilled water, and water plant B with a mild salt solution.
- Observe what happens to the two plants. Hypothesize about the reasons for their growth patterns, based on what you have learned about water movement in plants.

How Does Water Distribute Materials Within Animal Bodies?

JOB PROFILE: PHLEBOTOMIST

Sarah K. began working as a phlebotomist the day she turned 16 years old. "I had applied for jobs at the local hospital," she explains. "I got a call to come in at 5 am for a job with the hospital lab. The lady there explained to me that she wanted to train me as a phlebotomist, and she told me a phlebotomist takes people's blood. She talked to me about it; then she took my blood; then she had me take her blood. Then she sent me around the lab to take blood from all the lab workers. That was the beginning of my training. Now I've been at it for three years. I like it; I like the feeling that they depend on me."

Sarah goes on, "Blood is taken from patients for many different types of tests. Each group of tests has its own type of test tube. Tests are given to find antibodies to diseases, to find microbes, to type blood, to look at the blood cells to see if they're healthy, to check the levels of medication, all sorts of things."

"Usually I take blood from one of three main veins in the arm. If I can't find the vein there, I try the hands. I've taken blood from people's feet and even from veins in the scalps of babies."

"I like patients, going around meeting and talking with patients when I take their blood. And I like being financially independent."

All vertebrate animals (and many invertebrates as well) have circulatory systems. The human cardiovascular system is one type of circulatory system. It is a network of vessels through which blood is pumped by the heart (Figure 2-7). Blood carries nutrients to the body's cells and waste materials away from the cells. Blood is pumped away from the heart through arteries, then branches into smaller vessels called arterioles, and finally goes through a network of very narrow vessels not much wider than a red blood cell in diameter. These are called capillaries. While blood is in the capillaries, it exchanges various substances—gases, proteins, vitamins, salts, waste products—with the cells. These substances, along with water, pass through the highly permeable walls of the capillaries by diffusion. The direction in which they move is due, in part, to their concentration, both in the blood and in the tissues. Blood then enters a network of veins, smaller ones leading to larger ones until the blood goes back to the heart.

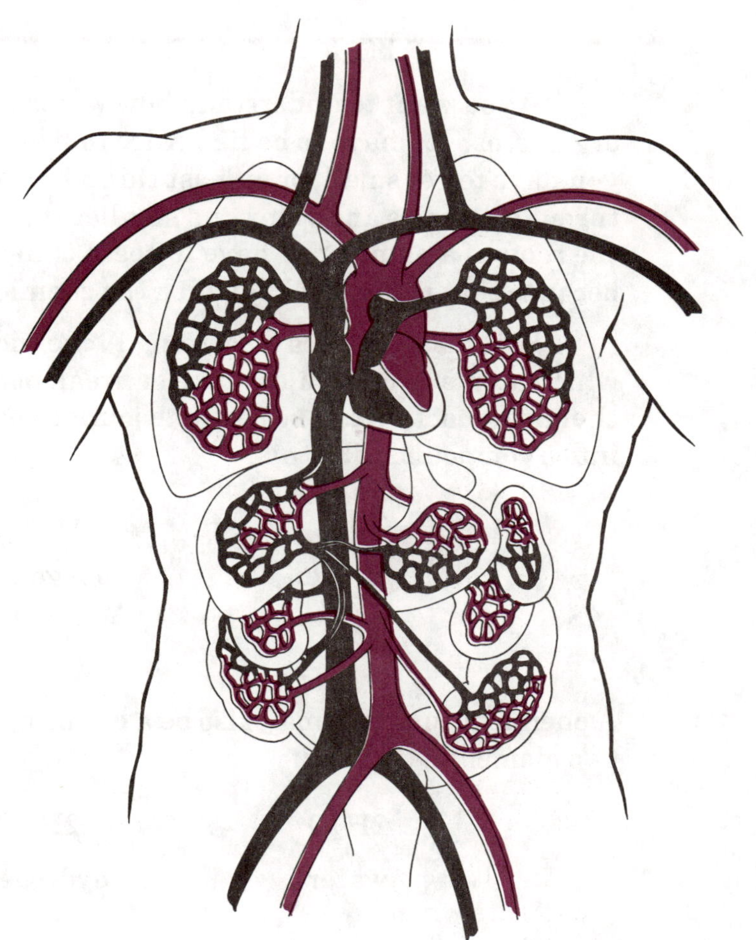

Figure 2-7 Human cardiovascular system

The vertebrate cardiovascular system is said to be closed. That is, there are no blood vessels that open into the body; all of them are connected to one another. However, in a real sense, the system is very open because it allows materials to move between the blood and the cells of other body tissues. This exchange takes place in the networks of capillaries.

One problem of a system that allows materials to move easily out of the blood is that more water is generally removed from the blood than is put back into it. For that reason, vertebrates also have a lymphatic system, an open circulatory system that gathers excess fluid from the body and drains it into the veins.

What Is the Role of Water in Biochemical Reactions?

If you want to understand how water functions inside organisms, you have to be like Alice in *Alice in Wonderland*. That is, you have to get small, or at least think small—smaller than bulk flow through arteries and veins and smaller than osmosis from the soil to the roots of a plant. You have to begin thinking on a molecular level because that is the level at which the chemical reactions take place.

What is a chemical reaction? A chemical reaction is an event in which atoms or molecules make or break bonds with each other. A chemical reaction can be a simple joining together of two elements into a compound, like this:

$2H_2$	+	O_2	→	$2H_2O$
hydrogen		oxygen		water

Equation 2-1

A chemical equation may also be a breaking apart of a compound into two elements, like this:

$2H_2O$	→	$2H_2$	+	O_2
water		hydrogen		oxygen

Equation 2-2

Some chemical reactions involve the regrouping of elements in two or more compounds, like this:

CH_4	+	$2O_2$	→	CO_2	+	H_2O
methane		oxygen		carbon dioxide		water

Equation 2-3

Substances that react in a chemical reaction are called the reactants. Substances produced by chemical reactions are called, as you might guess, products. In any chemical reaction, the number of atoms is the same before and after the reaction. That is, the number of atoms found in the reactants is the same as the number of atoms found in the product or products of that reaction. A chemical equation such as the ones in Equations 2-1, 2-2, and 2-3 reflects this. Thus, we say that these chemical equations are balanced. In other words, matter does not get lost in a chemical reaction. Energy may be absorbed or released, but the number of atoms stays the same.

Activity 2-7

In writing chemical equations, you must be sure that the number of atoms on each side of the equation is equal.

- Using the step-by-step procedure provided by your teacher, balance the equations below.

$$C_2H_6 + O_2 \rightarrow CO_2 + H_2O$$

$$CH_4 + O2 \rightarrow CO_2 + H_2O$$

$$C_4H_{10} + O_2 \rightarrow CO_2 + H_2O$$

- Compare your answers with those of students who sit next to you. If your answers are not the same, decide whose answers are correct and why.

What Are Biochemical Reactions?

Most of the functions of living organisms take place through a series of chemical reactions. A series of related chemical reactions occurring within an organism is called a *biochemical pathway*. In a biochemical pathway, the product of one step becomes the reactant of the next step. Respiration, photosynthesis, digestion, our very thought processes take place in sequential steps along biochemical pathways.

How Do Enzymes Affect Biochemical Reactions?

Another important aspect of biochemical pathways is the presence of enzymes. Enzymes are catalysts—substances that increase the rate of a chemical reaction but act as neither reactants nor products. A different enzyme acts as a catalyst for each step of a biochemical pathway. Enzymes increase reaction rates by many times what would occur spontaneously. For example, when carbon dioxide dissolves into the blood and is converted to carbonic acid, one enzyme molecule is working to convert nearly one million molecules of carbon dioxide to carbonic acid each second. If no enzyme were present the conversion rate would fall to less than one molecule per second!

How Do Biochemical Reactions Depend on Water?

Most of the biochemical reactions in the body occur in water. Water holds enzymes and reactants in solution. Water also holds a reservoir of positive and negative ions, available to enzymes for use in many reactions. Water helps to maintain a stable temperature in which reactions can take place. Water is often a reactant and a product somewhere along the sequence of steps that make up a biochemical pathway.

An example of a biochemical reaction that involves water is the process by which carbon dioxide leaves cells and enters the blood in vertebrate animals. In this reaction, water is one of the reactants. An enzyme called carbonic anhydrase is the catalyst in this reaction. It catalyzes the combination of carbon dioxide with water to form carbonic acid:

$$\underset{\text{carbon dioxide}}{CO_2} + \underset{\text{water}}{H_2O} \rightleftharpoons \underset{\text{carbonic acid}}{H_2CO_3}$$

Equation 2-4

The carbonic acid then breaks down into bicarbonate and hydrogen ions:

$$\underset{\text{carbonic acid}}{H_2CO_3} \rightleftharpoons \underset{\text{hydrogen ions}}{H^+} + \underset{\text{ionic bicarbonate}}{HCO_3^-}$$

Equation 2-5

By these two reactions, the concentration of carbon dioxide in the blood is lowered. The lower concentration of carbon dioxide in the blood causes additional carbon dioxide to diffuse into the blood from nearby tissue cells.

Water is a product of some biochemical pathways. Cellular respiration involves biochemical pathways composed of a long series of reactions. Water is one of the final products in this series, as shown in Equation 2-6:

$C(H_2O)$	+	$O_2 \rightarrow\rightarrow\rightarrow\rightarrow\rightarrow\rightarrow$	CO_2	+	H_2O
carbohydrate		oxygen	carbon dioxide		water

Equation 2-6

Activity 2-8

- The following equation summarizes a biochemical pathway in which water is a reactant. Based on what you know about plant processes, what process does it represent? Where do the reactants come from? What happens to the products?

$6H_2O$	+	$6CO_2$	$\rightarrow$	$C_6H_{12}O_6$	+	$6O_2$
water		carbon dioxide		sugar		oxygen

How Do Organisms Maintain Water Balance?

All organisms require water to maintain life, but they all have different needs when it comes to maintaining water balance. These needs vary with the organism's environment—land or water, arid land or moisture-rich land, salt water or fresh water. Also, as you might guess, animals and plants have very different problems to solve in order to maintain water balance.

Animal Water Balance

Most animals have in common certain mechanisms by which they maintain water balance. The diagram in Figure 2-8 shows how water gains and losses occur.

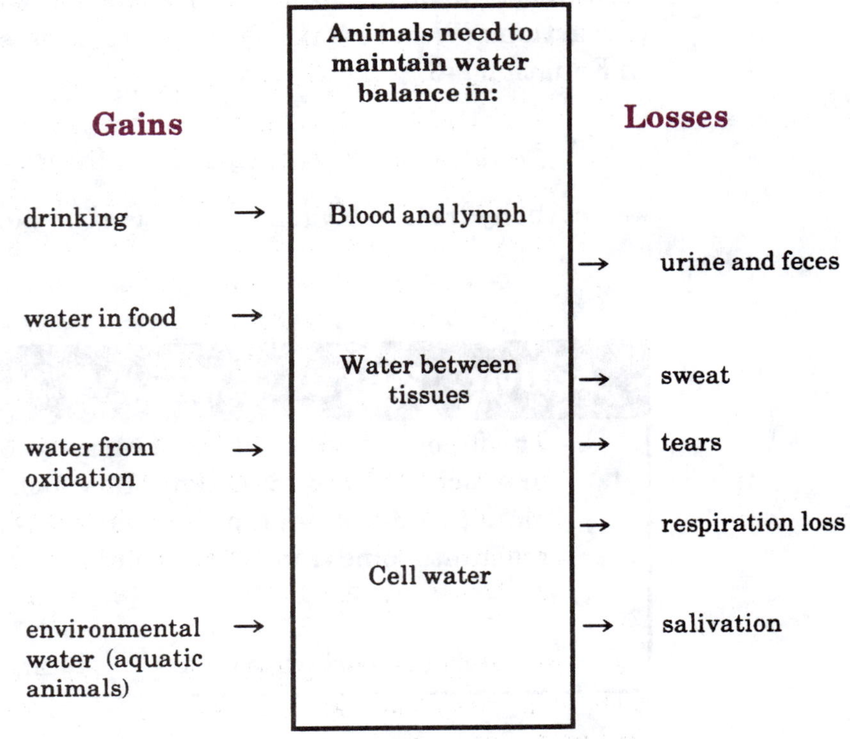

Figure 2-8 Schematic diagram of mechanisms of water gain and loss

For many animal species, the main water-balance problem is to find a way to get rid of the body's waste products without getting rid of all its water. To understand how animals retain body water, you have to understand the key process of osmosis. Recall from earlier in this subunit that osmosis is the diffusion of water across membranes, from an area of greater water concentration to an area of lesser water concentration.

Activity 2-9

Aquatic animals would seem to have no problem with water balance because they live in the water, but is this really so? In this activity, you can investigate water balance in two different types of aquatic environments: fresh water and salt water.

- Work in small groups. Based on what you have learned about osmosis, hypothesize about the water problems faced by freshwater and saltwater fish. Try to answer the questions: What is the main water problem faced by each group?
- Check the library to find out how accurate your group's ideas are. Report to the class on 1) your original hypothesis, 2) whether your thinking was correct or in error. 3) If your thinking was in error, analyze how your group went astray in your thinking.
- Do further research to learn how the water-regulating functions of freshwater and saltwater fish differ. For this portion of the activity, you may want to have one half the class investigate freshwater fish, one half investigate saltwater fish, and then compare your findings.

From the preceding activity, you can see the key role of osmosis in how fish get, keep, and rid themselves of water. Osmosis plays an important role in water retention for land animals, too. Some of the work of water reabsorption in vertebrate animals takes place in the filtering organ known as the kidney.

Here, we will focus on the human kidney as an example of vertebrate kidneys. The kidney is made up of about a million tiny tube (tubule) arrangements known as nephrons. A diagram of a kidney with an inset closeup of a nephron is shown in Figure 2-9. The nephrons are surrounded by kidney tissue that has a fairly high solute concentration.

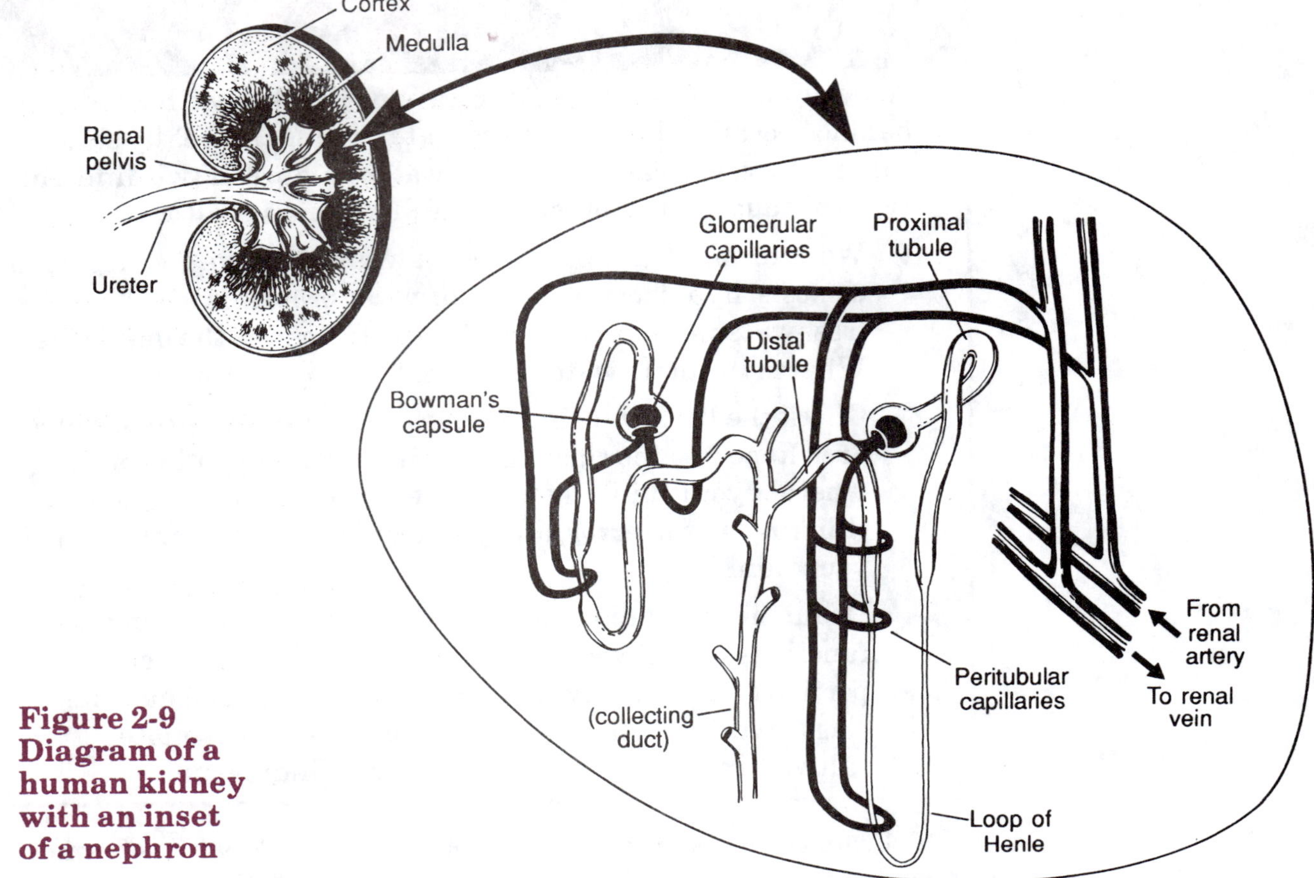

Figure 2-9 Diagram of a human kidney with an inset of a nephron

In general, the kidneys work by means of a series of changes in the solute concentration inside and outside of the nephron tubules. Differences in the solute concentration can cause the movement of water by osmosis. If body fluids are too dilute, the nephron tubules deliver water to the bladder as urine. But if the body is becoming dehydrated, the tubules lose water to the surrounding tissue by osmosis. This water is eventually reclaimed by the blood supply that serves the kidney. However, the function of the kidney is not dependent on osmosis alone. A system of active transport in the nephron tubules either excretes ions into the urine or passes them back to the blood, depending on the body's needs.

With so much attention to how animals retain water, we need to remember that the practical problem for human beings and other land animals is getting water in the first place. Unlike plants, animals can search for water when they need it. Animals kept as pets or raised for food consumption must rely on human caretakers to maintain their water supply. This can be a laborious task if you are working with many animals.

Activity 2-10

- Assume that you are going into the ranching business. You don't have a lot of experience, so you start off on a small scale. You buy a 150-acre ranch and 100 head of cattle. The land has no stock pond or tank to provide the herd with drinking water. The land is sandy in some areas and clayey in others. You know that the land has a natural spring as well as a plentiful underground water supply that you can tap. How can you best supply your herd with a year-round source of clean drinking water?
- Research your problem by talking to a local agricultural extension agent, animal husbandry teacher, or livestock veterinarian.
- Develop a plan or design for your solution.
- Share your solutions with the class. Discuss the solutions, their advantages and disadvantages. As a class, select two solutions that you think will work the best and be cost-effective.

Plant Water Balance

Unlike animals, plants are rooted in one location and must replenish their water supply fairly constantly. Plants respond very quickly to changes in water availability.

Greenscene

Greenscene, Inc. is a plant leasing and sales company. The owners, George S. and Malcolm L. started their business after taking horticulture classes at the local community college. They run the business together, but the responsibilities are divided. George directs everything to do with the plants; Malcolm is in charge of the financial side and oversees the building and maintenance of the greenhouses.

Recently Malcolm built the fourth greenhouse facility. He talks about how greenhouses contribute to plant water balance. "We use evaporative coolers to maintain adequate humidity," says Malcolm. "During the sunny days when the radiant heat is high, these swamp boxes do a good job. Humidity is a key factor in plant health, because if the plant intake of water does not keep up with the loss by evaporation, the plant starts to wilt. In our business, every plant delivered has to look in tip-top shape."

What measures does George take to maintain water balance in the plants he takes care of? George explains, "If you see a plant in trouble, you can mist it to cool the leaf surface and slow the rate of water loss. You can pull a shade over the top of the greenhouse to cut the radiant heat. If many plants are looking parched, I usually turn on the supplementary coolers and increase the humidity in the entire greenhouse."

Water balance in plants is affected by several processes: photosynthesis, transpiration, and osmosis. Each of these activities has an effect on the others. Photosynthesis cannot take place unless the stomata have been open to receive carbon dioxide. But open stomata result in water loss by transpiration. Water lost through transpiration is replaced by more water from the soil. Osmosis plays a major role in this uptake of water by developing root pressure. Root pressure occurs because of the solute difference between water inside the roots (greater solute concentration) and water in the soil (lower solute concentration).

The primary mechanism used by most plants to maintain water balance is the opening and closing of the stomata. The stomata are formed by cells known as guard cells. Water moves into the guard cells by osmosis whenever ion concentrations within those cells are high. Ion concentrations increase during the day when sunlight triggers an uptake of K^+ and Cl^- ions by the guard cells. This ion uptake is followed by movement of water into cells by osmosis, causing the cells to swell. When the guard cells are swollen with water, the stomata in between the cells are open. The plant is now in a condition in which it can afford to lose some water as it takes in carbon dioxide.

When the solute concentration in the guard cells is low, water moves back out of the guard cells and the stomata close. The plant cannot take in more carbon dioxide because it cannot afford to lose water.

Looking Back

Water makes up about two-thirds of the bodies of most vertebrates and is an important component of every organism on Earth for the following reasons. Water helps to regulate the body temperature of animals and plants because it has a high heat capacity and a high heat of vaporization.

Water is also an important transporter of nutrients and wastes in the body. Water moves inside the bodies of animals and plants partly by means of bulk flow. Two behaviors of water, diffusion and osmosis, play an important role in the transport of nutrients and other materials within organisms.

Water plays an important role in biochemical reactions in the body, holding enzymes and reactants in solution and maintaining a reservoir of positive and negative ions, available to enzymes for use when needed. Water is also often a reactant and a product in biochemical pathways, series of chemical reactions involved in life processes, such as respiration and photosynthesis.

Water balance is critical to the survival of animals and plants. The major challenge for land animals is to eliminate wastes without losing too much water. Most animals accomplish this, in large part, through the filtering organ known as the kidney. Plants replenish their water supply whenever water is available in the soil, bringing in water through the roots as it is lost through transpiration.

Further Discussion

- Many animals do not form urine, thereby greatly reducing their water losses. Insects, reptiles and birds, for instance, eliminate part of their waste products in the form of a white, pasty material (called uric acid) that contains very little water. Select one of the above three groups and discuss the reasons you feel would explain the need for this special adaptation in that group.
- You learned in this unit that capillaries are very narrow blood vessels across which substances pass between blood and tissues. But what determines in which direction (into or out of the blood) a given substance will move? Discuss the importance of all factors you feel are involved in capillary exchange. (Remember

that, apart from other forces, the blood is under pressure from the beating of the heart.)

- Some organisms have non-wettable tissues. Some examples are the waxy leaves of some aquatic plants and the feathers of ducks. Find out how these surfaces resist water and why such resistance to water is necessary for the organisms involved

Activities by Occupational Area

General

Water Balance in Aquatic Animals

- Visit a marina, a tropical fish store, or an aquarium maintained by a company or institution.
- Select one type of fish or other aquatic animal kept there and talk to its caretaker.
- Find out the following:
  1. How does this organism take in water?
  2. How does it get rid of water?
- Report your findings to the class.

Rehydrating the Body

- Athletes and workers whose jobs cause them to sweat a great deal have to continually replenish the water in their bodies to prevent dehydration. The best way to do this has been the subject of controversy. Some say that drinking plain water is best while others maintain that a sports drink that contains glucose and electrolytes is better.
- Research the issue by talking to sports trainers, athletes, and medical professionals and/or through library research.
- Summarize the views of proponents of each side. Which arguments are most convincing to you?

Agriculture and Agribusiness

Effects of Soil Type on Water Availability

- Investigate the effects of soil type on the availability of water to plants by consulting with a landscape gardener or landscape architect.
- Find out what kinds of plants grow well in the soil type around your school or home.

Cost-Effectiveness of Raising Animals for Food in Arid Regions

- Assume you are from an arid region of the country. You are interested in raising some type of animal to be sold as food.
- Investigate what animals are easiest to raise on arid lands. Select the animal of your choice and explain to the class why you chose this animal.

  Please note: If the animal of your choice is not part of the typical American diet, you need to come up with a marketing plan for selling it as food.

Health Occupations

Fever as an Indicator of Illness

- An important part of a nurse's job is to monitor the vital signs of a patient. Vital signs include body temperature, blood pressure, and pulse.
- Interview a nurse to find out why body temperature is such an important indicator of a patient's condition. Ask for examples of situations in which the patient's body temperature provides important information about his or her condition.
- Report your findings to the class.

Drowning

- Talk to an emergency medical technician (EMT) or emergency room doctor about drowning. Have him or her discuss the differences in drowning in fresh water and in salt water.
- Find the answers to the following questions:
  1. What happens to the victim in each type of drowning?
  2. What effect does water temperature have in the drowning?
  3. How does emergency treatment differ for each type of patient?

Home Economics

Quality of Bottled Waters

- Investigate the quality of bottled waters currently on the market. You will need to use the *Reader's Guide to Periodical Literature*. You may wish to check *Consumer Reports*.
- Answer the following questions:
    1. How are bottled waters checked for contaminants?
    2. What are the differences among bottled waters?
    3. Are some bottled waters considered by doctors and nutritionists to be healthier than others? If so, which ones?

Industrial Technology

Reverse Osmosis

- Contact a water-purification company that uses the process of reverse osmosis.
- Find out how reverse osmosis is being applied. Compare these applications to osmosis in living systems.

LAB 1

MOVEMENT OF MOLECULES ACROSS A MEMBRANE

PREVIEW

Introduction

Dr. E. is a doctor who directs a pediatric intensive care unit. Among the many different medical procedures that he carries out in the unit is one called peritoneal dialysis.

Peritoneal dialysis is used to cleanse the blood of excess salts and waste products when the kidneys are not functioning properly. "In peritoneal dialysis," Dr. E. explains, "the body's peritoneal cavity [the space between the inner and outer layers of the sac lining the abdominal walls] is used as one side of a semipermeable membrane. The other side is the capillary bed of the walls of the intestine. The idea is to rid the blood of waste products by equilibrating it with the fluid on the other side in the cavity." The cavity is flooded with a solution, which changes the osmotic gradient, causing waste products to cross the membrane into the cavity, where they can be sucked out along with excess water. The main solute used in the solution is sugar.

"This procedure is used in case of renal failure," explains Dr. E. However, with children, we use it more often to treat acidosis that is caused by an infection or by poor cardiac output."

Purpose

In this lab, you will determine the effect of concentration difference on the movement of water and solute across a membrane.

Lab Objective

When you've finished this lab, you will be able to—

- Predict the direction of material movement across a membrane based on the concentration of materials on both sides of the membrane.

Lab Skills

You will use these skills to complete this lab—

- Measure mass with a triple-beam balance.
- Prepare and fill dialysis bags.

Materials and Equipment Needed

4 pieces of dialysis tubing 6 inches long

string

triple-beam balance

marking pencil

4 quart jars or 500-ml beakers

1 liter of distilled water

100 ml of 5% NaCl solution

100 ml of 10% NaCl solution

1 liter of 15% NaCl solution

LAB PROCEDURE

Pre-Lab Discussion

The removal of waste from the blood is normally the job of the kidneys. However, sometimes due to injury or disease, the kidneys do not adequately do this job. When this happens, toxic materials such as creatinine and urea build up in the blood. This condition is a serious life-threatening situation. Unless something is done a person can die from kidney failure. One method of treating this condition is called peritoneal dialysis. The dialysis fluid is put into the peritoneal cavity in the abdomen. The dialysis fluid bathes the intestines and other organs in the abdomen with a solution that has a low concentration of urea and creatinine. These materials move from the blood into the dialysis fluid. After a few hours, the dialysis fluid is drained and the urea and creatinine are removed from the body.

In this lab, you will look at how salt and water move across a dialysis membrane. This movement gets material into and out of cells. It also can have a drastic effect on fish and other aquatic animals and plants if they are moved from a habitat with a high salt concentration to a habitat with a low salt concentration, or vice versa.

Method

Put on your lab apron and goggles.

1. Label each beaker with one of the following labels:

   5% NaCl in H_2O
   10% NaCl in H_2O
   15% NaCl in H_2O
   H_2O in 15% NaCl

2. Soak six pieces of string in distilled water and two pieces of string in 15% NaCl.
3. Prepare dialysis bags by tying one end of each section of tubing as shown in Figure L1-1.

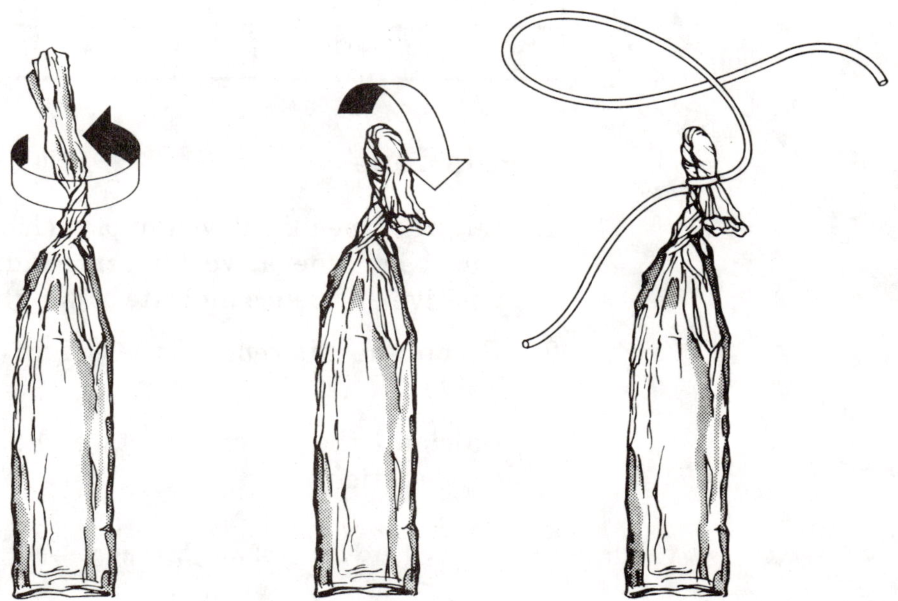

Figure L1-1 Tying the end of a dialysis bag

4. Each bag should be timed independently and the timing staggered by four to five minutes. Do the following for each bag.
   - Fill each bag with one of the NaCl solutions (5%, 10%, or 15%) or with water to within 1 to 2 inches of the top end.
   - Tie the open end of the bag so that the bag is limp (the bag should have room for more liquid).
   - Dry and weigh the bag.
   - Record this initial weight of the bag in the Data Table.
   - Place each bag in the appropriately labeled beaker or jar.

5. Fill each beaker or jar with either water or 15% NaCl as indicated on the label.
6. As 30 minutes elapse for each bag, remove the bag from the beaker or jar, dry the bag, weigh the dried bag, and record the final weight of the bag in the Data Table.

Data Table

Bag	Final Weight	Initial Weight	Weight Difference
5% NaCl in H_2O			
10% NaCl in H_2O			
15% NaCl in H_2O			
H_2O in 15% NaCl			

Calculations

1. Subtract the initial weight of each bag from the final weight of each bag. A negative difference indicates a weight loss and a positive difference indicates a weight gain.
2. Record the difference in the weight of each bag in the Data Table.
3. Calculate the percentage of weight difference for each bag using the equation:

$$\text{Percentage of weight change} = \frac{\text{Weight difference}}{\text{Initial weight}} \times 100$$

4. Graph concentration of solute in bag versus percentage of weight change.

Cleanup Instructions

- Empty the solutions from the beakers and dialysis bags into the sink.
- Throw the emptied dialysis bags in the trash.
- Wash the beakers and return them to their proper location.

WRAP-UP

Conclusions

1. Which bag(s) had the largest weight change?
2. In which direction did the material apparently travel through the membrane in each bag?
3. In peritoneal dialysis, would you expect the solute concentration of the dialysis fluid to be greater than or less than the solute concentration in the body fluids.
4. Explain the direction in which the material apparently traveled across the membrane for each bag.

Challenge Questions and Extensions

5. Based on your data, what would happen to the body fluids of a marine fish in a fresh water lake?
6. Based on your data, what would happen to the body fluids of a fresh water fish in the Atlantic Ocean?

SUBUNIT 3

How Is Water Used?

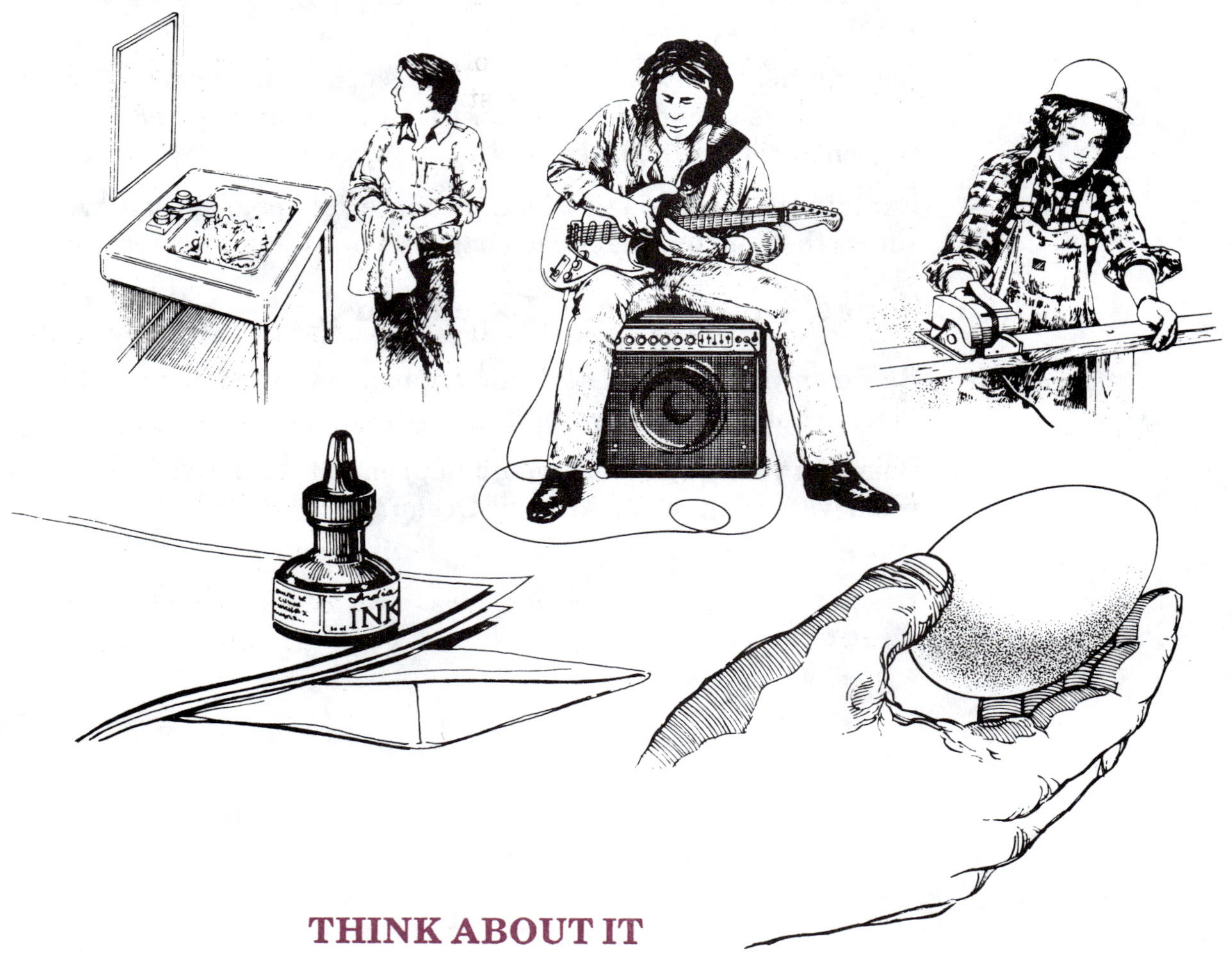

THINK ABOUT IT

- Each picture above represents an object or a service that requires water to produce. How do you think that water is used in the production of each object or service?
- Which item or service do you think uses the most water for its production? Try to rank order the five pictures from the one that represents the greatest water use to the one that represents the least water use.
- If the water supply were limited, which items or service would you rank as most important and which as least important?

SUBUNIT OBJECTIVES

After you complete this subunit, you will be able to —

1. Assess the impact on water quantity of use by different sectors of society: domestic, industrial, and agricultural.
2. Identify at least four functions of water in industry and link those functions to specific industries.
3. Explain how hydrogen bonding affects water's function as a solvent.
4. Give examples of the "like dissolves like" rule in the everyday use of solutions.
5. Create an advertisement that illustrates the way that soap aids water in dissolving nonpolar solutes.
6. Determine the amounts of solute required for solutions of various concentrations, using three different types of units: molar, normal and percent composition, as appropriate.
7. Calculate dilution to a desired concentration.
8. Describe at least three occupations in which a knowledge of solutions is needed.

What Are the Competing Demands for Water?

Hondo Springs, continued

Leroy Davis and Veronica Garcia sit at a coffee shop across the street from City Hall. They have just been to see Councilmember Carol Overby to talk about the controversy over Hondo Springs. "Well, at least we got in to see her," says Veronica, dipping a French fry in a puddle of ketchup, "even if we didn't get that much real information."

"Maybe we got too much information," replies Leroy, munching on his burger. "But we don't like it because it doesn't fit with our opinion."

"What do you mean, our opinion?" asks Veronica indignantly. "I haven't formed any opinion yet; I'm still getting information!"

"Oh, come on, Veronica. You know we've both been leaning against development of the recharge zone ever since we went to the springs with Ms. Li to do the life-form survey. Anybody who hangs out at Hondo Springs and sees how peaceful and nice it is, is bound to start wondering if the city should let anybody mess with it."

"Well, okay, I guess I'm not completely objective," admits Veronica. "It's confusing to hear Overby's opinion. She makes it sound like we're going to be a ghost town if we don't develop that recharge zone."

"But the real question is, will the development destroy the springs? Because that would hurt the town, too. She says the fecal coliform count has always been high at the springs, that the recent increases don't mean anything. And what about what she says about the high-tech industries being 'clean industries'? Do you think it's true?"

Veronica sits up decisively. "I don't know, but we need more than her opinion. We need facts about who uses the water and how the runoff is affected. We don't know what kind of land use is likely to pollute the springs and what kind might be pretty harmless. We don't know how water is used in industry at all!"

"Where do we get that kind of information?" asks Leroy.

"A lot of it is right across the street at City Hall. Some of it is probably at the City Water Department. And I'll bet some of it might be at the local office of the Environmental Protection Agency. Don't worry, we'll find it. It just takes a little investigative work."

"Doesn't sound like a little anything to me. It sounds like all my free time for the next two months," Leroy grumbles. But when he sees the disappointed look on Veronica's face, he says quickly, "but I can handle it. Don't worry, you can count me in!"

Water has long been associated with commerce. The production of crops and livestock has always been dependent upon the availability of water. Cities often have been built beside rivers partly because the rivers provided a means of transporting products to and from other places. Beginning in this century, water provided a source of power for the production of electricity used to run factories and supply homes. In industry, water is often used as a coolant, a transporter of materials, a lubricant, or a product ingredient.

How much water does it take to produce energy, to grow crops and raise domestic animals, to carry out industrial processes and to maintain sanitation and personal hygiene? In other words, what are the competing uses of water in a developed society?

Activity 3-1

- In a small group, develop a brief questionnaire to find out how much the class already knows about water use. Include questions about the following:
  - the percentage of water use in each of these categories–agriculture, industry, domestic use, and recreational use
  - the effect of different uses on water quality
  - the effect of different uses on water quantity
- Administer your survey and compile the results. Present the results to the class.
- Save the questionnaires and the survey results for use later on in this unit.

Water use is roughly estimated to be divided among agriculture, industry and domestic uses as shown in Table 3-1. We will look briefly at each type of use.

Table 3-1: Estimated Worldwide Water Use (1985)

Domestic uses	7%
Industrial uses	23%
Agricultural uses	70%

Domestic Use of Water

Domestic use of water includes water used for drinking and cooking, bathing and personal hygiene, washing dishes and clothes, and flushing toilets (Figure 3-1).

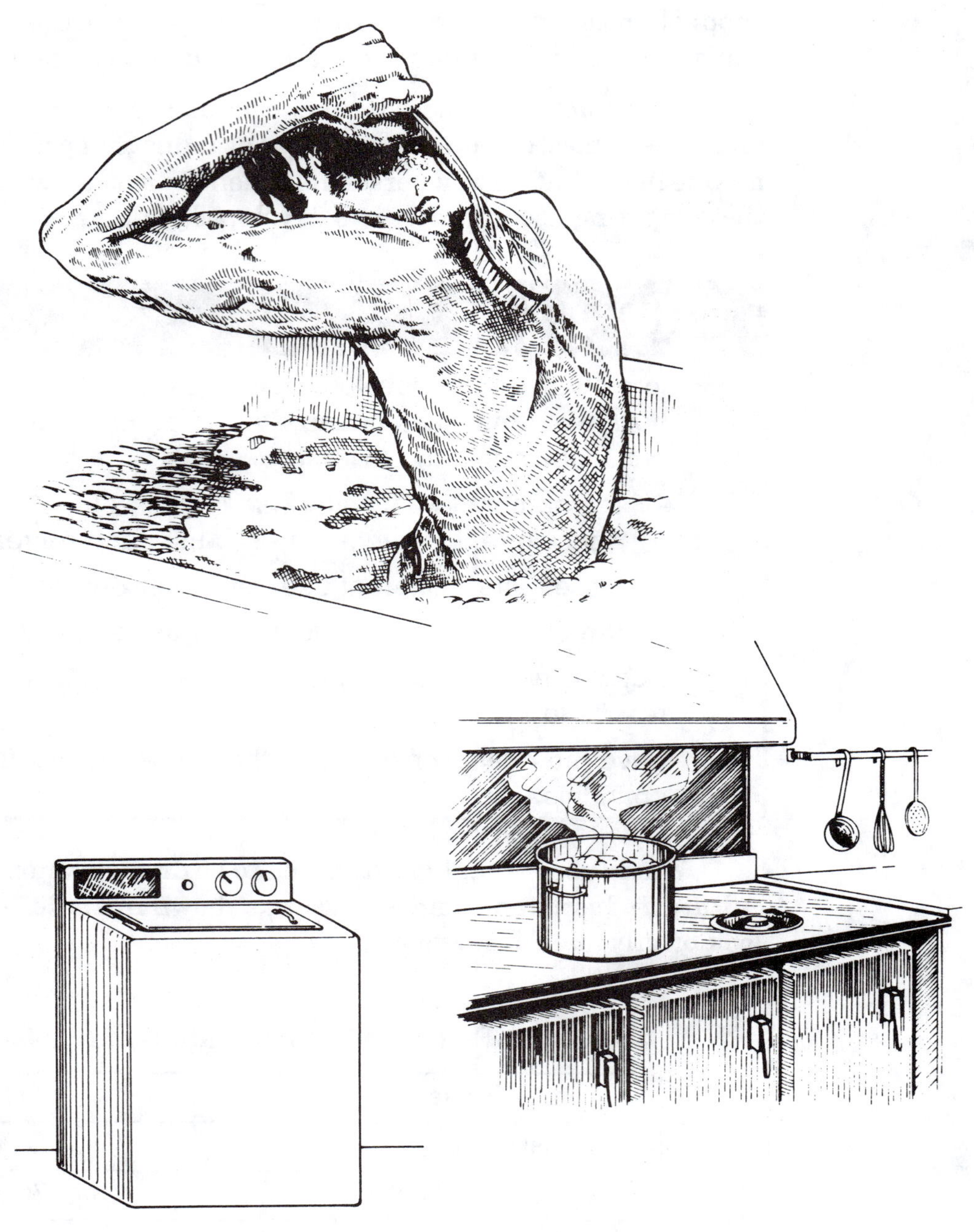

Figure 3-1 Domestic uses of water

It is estimated that about 50 gallons (190 liters) of water are needed per person per day to maintain the generally accepted minimum standards of sanitation and grooming in this society. Table 3-2 shows how the fifty gallons might be divided.

Table 3-2: How To Survive on 50 Gallons [190 Liters] of Water per Person per Day

Use	What It Uses	Water Budget	Percent Used
Toilet	5-7 gal (9-27 liters) per flush	15 gal (54 liters) for 3 flushes	30
Dishwashing	20 gal (76 liters) per load for automatic; 5-10 gal (18-38 liters) if by hand	10 gal (38 liters)	20
Shower	3 gal/min (11 liters/min)	9 gal (34 liters)	18
Tub	25-30 gal (95-114 liters)	Don't use	
Hygiene	3 gal/min to run tap. (11 liters/min)	9 gal (34 liters)	18
Clothes washing	30-40 gal per load (114-152 liters)	5 gal (wash once per week) (19 liters)	10
Other	2 gal/drinking, cooking, watering, other (8 liters)	2 gal (8 liters)	4

Source: N.J. Department of Environmental Protection, 1985.

Actual domestic use of water varies quite a lot. In urban households with piped-in water, daily use ranges between 100 and 350 liters (26-92 gallons) per person per day. In homes equipped with dishwashers, washing machines, and outdoor sprinkler systems, consumption may reach 1000 liters (264 gallons) per person per day.

Activity 3-2

- Keep a water-use log for two days. You will need the cooperation of your family because some of your water use is shared, such as water used to do the family's dishes or clothes.
- Post small charts or notepads and pencils in appropriate places to collect information: outside the bathroom, above the kitchen sink, beside the washing machine and dishwasher (if you have these). Ask your family to estimate how much water they used for different activities (example: five-minute shower, one minute of running tap for brushing teeth, etc.) Ask each family member to make a check mark on the record sheet for each time they flush the toilet.

- Compile the information after two full days. Estimate your family's per person per day average water use.
- In your ABC notebook, compare the data you collected with the uses shown in Table 3-2 to answer the following questions:
  - Is your family's per person per day average higher or lower than the 50-gallon (190 liters) rate in the table?
  - How does your family use the most water? In what activity, if any, does your family appear to use less water than that shown in the table?
  - Do your data change your ideas about domestic water use?
  - How did your family members react to having their water consumption monitored?

Agricultural Use of Water

The primary agricultural use of water is for irrigation. Irrigation allows farmers to get higher yields (more crops per acre) from the land under cultivation. Drip irrigation, in which water is applied directly to each plant rather than sprinkled on an entire field under cultivation, has proven to be an efficient delivery system, especially in dry regions (Figure 3-2). Depending on their location, farmers may obtain irrigation water from surface water sources, or they may have to pump from groundwater. Surface water costs tend to be lower for farmers. Pumping groundwater can be expensive, depending on the depth of the groundwater and the cost of fuel for pumping. Farmers also have to bear the cost of distributing water to the fields.

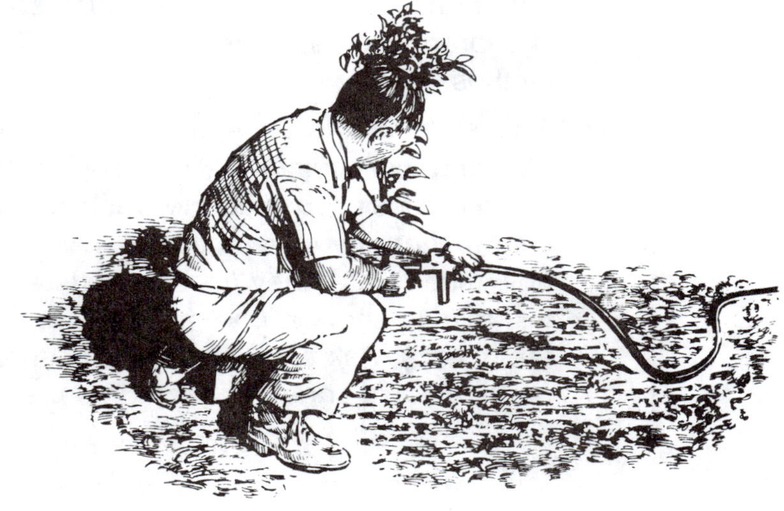

Figure 3-2 Drip irrigation system delivers water to each plant

It is estimated that in the U.S. about 55% of water withdrawn for agricultural use is consumed. That is, it is used up and cannot be returned to the stream or aquifer from which it is withdrawn. Some of that 55% is used up by crops. However, more water is delivered to the crop than the crops actually use. Other agricultural activities also consume water.

Activity 3-3

- In small groups, hypothesize about factors that could account for some of the water that is withdrawn for agricultural purposes but not returned to its source.
- Conduct research by consulting library sources, farmers, or agricultural advisors (extension agents, college professors).
- Decide, as a group, whether your hypotheses were realistic (not necessarily true or untrue, but realistic).
- Develop an experimental strategy for testing one or more of your hypotheses.

Besides irrigation, farmers use water for raising livestock. In recent years, aquaculture businesses have become major water consumers. Some aquaculture businesses use existing surface waters as the habitat for their fish or seafood. Others pump from an underground aquifer to fill tanks constructed especially for the purpose of raising aquatic species.

Catfish Business Meets State Regulation

Nat M. is a catfish farmer, and until recently business has been very good, so good that he has been able to build a total of 52 tanks for raising catfish. Where does he get the water to fill the 52 tanks? He pumps it—all 43 million gallons a day needed to operate his farm—from the aquifer below his land. After five years in operation, his facilities are in great shape, sales are terrific, but Nat has a very big problem.

The 43 million gallons of water per day is part of the problem. A nearby university town points out that Nat's farm uses more than 6 times the water used by all their residents and businesses combined. During a recent dry period, water levels in the aquifer dropped to the point that water rationing was imposed on the whole town, and some of the residents blame the catfish farm. It isn't as if Nat has been breaking the law by pumping water out of the aquifer. Until last week, there were no permit requirements. But complaints about the farm mounted, and state legislators finally acted to require permits for aquaculture businesses drawing water out of the aquifer. Nat has a little over a month to obtain a permit. He isn't sure what the result of the permit procedure will be. Will the state require him to pay a fee for the water? Will they limit his usage?

If Nat's only problem were water usage, he might not be so worried. But he has another problem. The state's water commission and the regional water authorities have been testing the water that is discharged from the catfish farm into a nearby lake. Nat holds in his hand a letter from the state agency informing him that they have detected heavy levels of fecal coliform bacteria in the discharge. The letter gives Nat 15 days to outline a plan to reduce or eliminate pollution from the discharge and about 20 additional days to carry out the plan.

Nat feels like the state is out to get him. His attitude is, "This is my land and I can take as much water from it as I need. I've worked hard to make this business, and no one has a right to limit the amount of money I can make." As far as the pollution is concerned, he figures that he can find a way to treat the discharge, and he plans to do it, but the time limit seems unfair to him. "These state bureaucrats don't understand what it's like to run a business," he says to himself.

Activity 3-4

- As a class, discuss Nat's attitude about the problems he is having with the state. Do you agree or disagree with his belief that he should be able to use as much water as he needs?
- Assume you are a partner in Nat's catfish farm. How are you going to respond publicly to the state's demands for a permit and a reduction of pollution in the farm's discharge water? Whom do you need to consult? What steps do you need to take? Make a plan of action.
- Compare your plan to that of others in the class.

Industry Use of Water

As shown in Table 3-1, industrial use of water accounts for about 23% of total water use, worldwide. However, in the U.S., water use in industry slightly exceeds its use in agriculture. In many other highly industrialized countries also, industry's percent of total water use is high. In England, for example, industry uses almost 70% of the water withdrawn from surface and groundwater. Contrast that with the industry water use of less than 10% in Mexico!

The leading industry use of water is in the production of electricity from fossil-fueled and nuclear power plants. Water is converted to steam to drive the turbines, and water is used as a coolant in power-plant condensers. Besides the use of water in power production, water is consumed in the mining and transport of fossil fuels. For example, coal is often transported in a slurry, a mixture of solid coal and water that is carried through a pipeline. Water is also lost in the process of mining, especially surface mining, and is required to restore land that has been surface-mined to a usable condition.

Water is used in other industries in several different ways: as a coolant, as a transporter of materials, as a lubricant, or as a product ingredient. Five industries use about two-thirds of all water used by industry. The chemical industry leads the way, followed closely by primary metals such as steel, then paper products, petroleum and coal refining, and food processing. Other industries that use 1% to 2% of the total industry water withdrawals include stone, clay and glass; nonelectrical and electrical machinery and equipment; rubber, lumber and wood products; textiles; and transportation.

Activity 3-5

- Select one of the industry categories listed in the paragraph above. Investigate that industry's use of water by interviewing a company or industry representative or by using library sources.
- Present your information to the class.
- As a class, develop a matrix of industry water use that lists types of industries and the functions of water in those industries: coolant, transporter of materials, lubricant, ingredient, etc.
- As a class, hypothesize about which industries are likely to have the greatest impact on water quantity and water quality.

By now, you are probably beginning to get an idea of the many commercial uses of water. These commercial uses, especially the uses of water in industry, are the focus of this subunit. But, to understand these industrial processes, you need to know more about water chemistry. In the rest of the subunit and the next one, we will examine two aspects of water chemistry that play an important role in its industrial uses: water's function as a solvent and the acid-base chemistry of water.

How Does Water Dissolve Material?

Many of the uses of water in industry are dependent on the use of water in solutions. A solution is a **homogeneous** mixture of two or more materials. Homogeneous means the mixture is the same throughout. In order for materials to mix, one of the materials must interrupt the forces that hold the molecules of the other substance together. This process is called **dissolving**.

The parts of a solution are the solvent and the solute. The **solvent** is the part of the solution that makes up the larger portion of the solution. It is usually a liquid, but it can be a solid or gas. The solvent is the material that interrupts the forces that hold the molecules of the other substance, the solute, together. Therefore, a solvent is a substance that can dissolve another substance.

The **solute** is the material that makes up the smaller portion of the solution. The solute can be a solid, liquid or a gas. Therefore, a solute is a substance that is dissolved in another substance.

How Does the Molecular Structure of Water Make It a Good Solvent?

Water is used as an ingredient or component of products in the pharmaceutical industry, in the food processing industry, in the cosmetics industry and in the chemical industry. Water is a key ingredient in many products of these industries because it is such a good solvent for many materials.

Water is able to dissolve material because of its molecular structure. Let's look again at the molecular structure of water. As you learned in Subunit 1, a water molecule is formed of one oxygen molecule that shares electrons with each of two hydrogen atoms. Because the nucleus of the oxygen atom pulls harder on the shared electrons than the hydrogen does, the oxygen atoms have a slightly negative charge. The hydrogen atoms, with their electrons drawn away somewhat, have a slightly positive charge. Thus we say that water is a polar molecule.

The **polarity** of water molecules causes them to cling to each other to some extent. The negative end of one water molecule is attracted to the positive end of another water molecule, and so on. These attractions are called **hydrogen bonds**. Compared to other kinds of chemical bonds, these are weak attractions. However, taken all together, the hydrogen bonds in a quantity of water have enough strength that they cannot be broken without a great deal of energy (Figure 3-3).

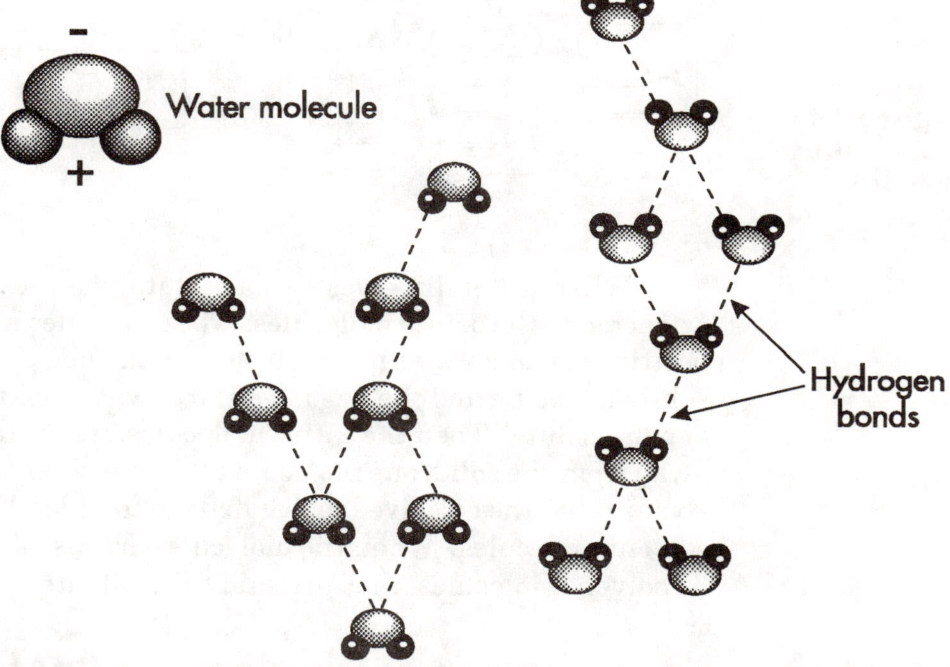

Figure 3-3 Hydrogen bonding of water

Activity 3-6

- Work in pairs for this activity. Get 12 red gum drops, 24 green gumdrops and a box of toothpicks from your teacher.
- Use the red gumdrops to represent oxygen, the green gumdrops to represent hydrogen and the toothpicks to represent covalent bonds within molecules. Arrange the gumdrops to represent 12 identical models of the water molecule. Use Figure 1-7 as a guide.
- Arrange the 12 models to represent hydrogen bonds among water molecules. Use an appropriate material to show that hydrogen bonds are weaker than covalent bonds.

Because water is a polar molecule, the solutes that can dissolve in water usually are also polar. How does water dissolve these materials? Let's consider a polar solute that is solid. In the solid state, the polar molecules align so that the negative end of one molecule is next to the positive end of another molecule (Figure 3-4).

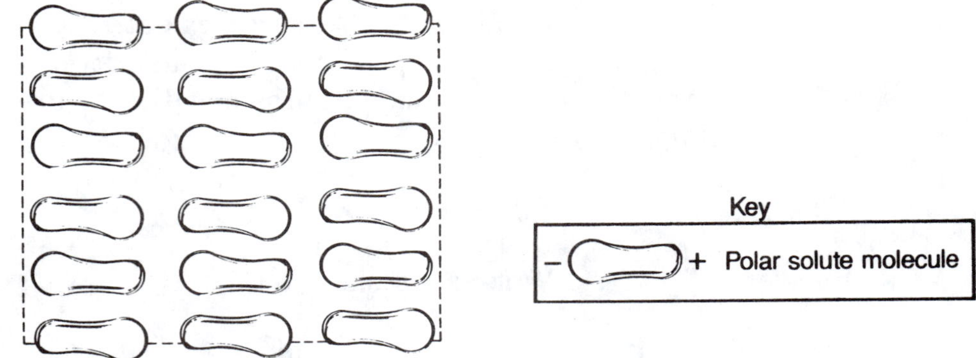

Figure 3-4 Polar solute in solid form

When water dissolves a polar solute, the water molecules are attracted to the solute molecules. The molecules align with the positive end of a water molecule next to the negative end of a polar solute molecule and the negative end of water next to the positive end of polar solute. Then the water molecules break the solute molecules away from the solid, one molecule at a time, as shown in Figure 3-5. Eventually, the dissolved molecules are completely surrounded by solvent molecules. When the molecules are dissolved and surrounded by solvent molecules, they are said to be solvated.

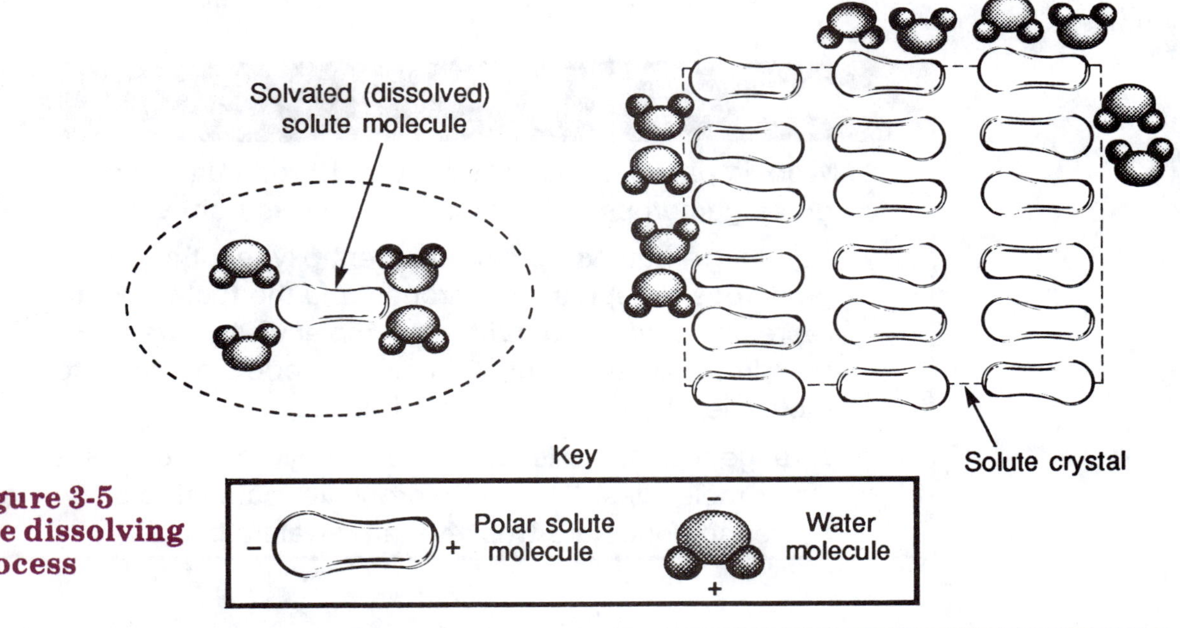

Figure 3-5 The dissolving process

“Like Dissolves Like” Rule

Besides being a component of many products, water is used as a solvent in many industrial processes. Water is used especially to remove unwanted materials from a raw material or final product. However, water is not the only solvent used in this way. Many other solvents exist and are used for various purposes. Mineral spirits is a solvent used for oil-based paints. Acetone is a solvent for many synthetic polymers (plastics).

Have you ever tried to use water to clean a paintbrush used for an oil-based paint? If you have, you know that water does not work as a solvent with such paints. Why is that so? What determines which solvent will dissolve which solute?

Activity 3-7

- Conduct a simple investigation of the ability of water to act as a solvent. Apply smudges of various types of cosmetics (waterproof and regular) to the back of your own hand.
- Attempt to remove these smudges using water as a solvent. How well does water work as a solvent for this purpose?

Like water, many solvents are **polar**. That is, there is a slight separation of charges in the molecule of the solvent resulting in one end of the molecule that is positive and one end that is negative. Many solute materials are also polar. Polar solvents will dissolve polar solutes.

Other solutes are **nonpolar**. That means the molecule either has no separation of charges, or the molecule has a symmetry that is the same on both sides of the center of the molecules. The symmetry causes separation of charges to balance out around the center of the molecule. Nonpolar solutes will dissolve nonpolar molecules.

A simple test to determine if a compound is polar or nonpolar is to try to dissolve the compound in several solvents, some polar and some nonpolar. Polar compounds will dissolve in polar solvents, and nonpolar compounds will dissolve in nonpolar solvents. You may have often heard that oil and water do not mix. That is because oil is nonpolar and water is polar. A chemical rule of thumb is that “like dissolves like.” Can you think of some experiences that you have had with household substances or foods that would seem to verify the “like dissolves like” rule?

How Does Soap Aid Water in the Dissolving Process?

If water does not mix with oil, you may ask, how is it that water is so often used for cleaning? After all, we wash dirty laundry with oil stains in water, not in mineral spirits. What happens to the "like dissolves like" rule in the washing machine?

It is true that water is not a good solvent for nonpolar solutes such as oil or grease. And in washing, much of the dirt that needs to be cleaned is nonpolar. It takes soap to aid water in dissolving the nonpolar dirt.

What is soap? Soap is the salt of a strong base (a base is a substance that forms hydroxide ions when it is mixed with water) such as sodium hydroxide (NaOH) and a long-chain fatty acid. The fatty acid consists of a long hydrocarbon chain (from 10 to 20 carbon units long) with a carboxylic acid group at one end. Figure 3-6 shows the process by which soap is made. The combination of the fatty acid and the sodium hydroxide yields water and a sodium salt, which is the soap.

When the soap dissolves in water, the sodium ion can be easily removed from the salt, leaving the negative ion of the fatty acid. This end of the fatty acid is the polar end of the soap molecule. The ionized soap molecule thus has a long nonpolar hydrocarbon "tail" and the polar, negatively charged "head" where the sodium ion used to be. In a water solution, these molecules form **micelles** (spheres with nonpolar tails pointed to the inside of the sphere and the charged heads on the surface). Why do you think that they organize themselves in this way?

The soap forms micelles because the nonpolar "tail" repels the water and the negatively charged "head" attracts the water. Nonpolar dirt can dissolve in the micelle and mix with the tails of the soap molecules. This process is shown in Figure 3-6.

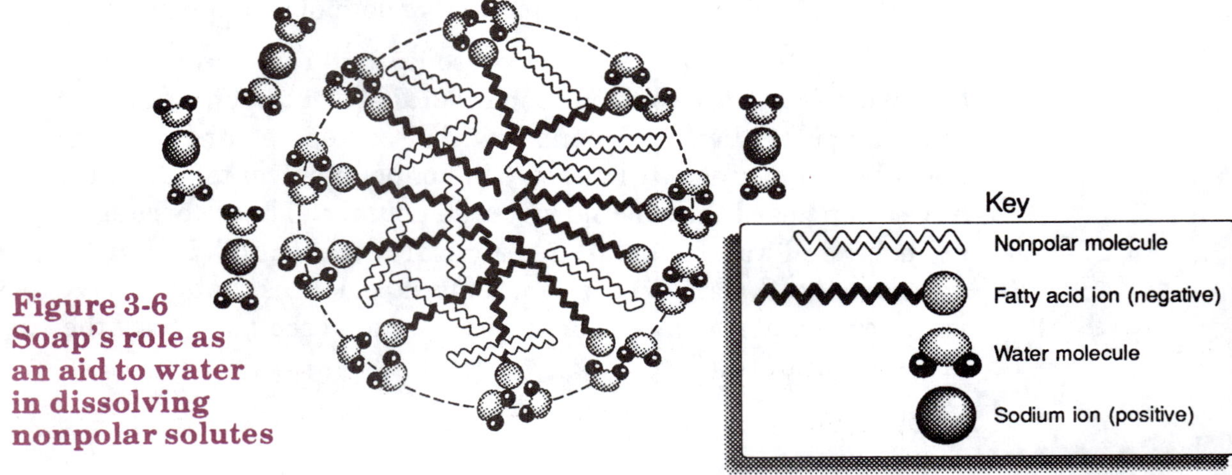

Figure 3-6 Soap's role as an aid to water in dissolving nonpolar solutes

Soap and detergents are used not only to do dishes and laundry in the home, but also to clean industrial materials. Textiles, pulp and paper, and other manufacturing activities involve the use of a soap or detergent at some stage of processing.

Activity 3-8

- In small groups, create a storyboard for a commercial advertising an imaginary soap product. Develop your commercial as you wish, but you must include the formation of micelles as part of your sales pitch.
- Share your storyboard with the rest of the class.

  Remember: Your drawings for the storyboard do not have to be highly developed. They should be diagrams. You can use stick figures and other simplified forms to get your idea across clearly.

How Is the Concentration of Solutions Measured?

Condition Red!

Yvonne Ybarra is having an off-day at the textile plant, no, make that an off-week. Her job is to monitor the water quality of all of the water used in the plant's production processes. She also oversees the quality of water released by the plant into the nearby river; this outgoing water is known as effluent.

Yvonne has to make regular reports to the Environmental Protection Agency (EPA) and other government agencies. However, these agencies don't just take Yvonne's word for it when it comes to water quality; they also monitor the quality of the river water at regular intervals.

This week Yvonne has a quarterly report due to the EPA; she also has some reports to make to the plant manager. So the last thing she needs is a complication, but that's just what she's got. The plant effluent is showing a higher concentration of residual dye than is acceptable to return to the river. The effluent meets EPA standards, but it doesn't meet state standards or the plant's own standard of an acceptable concentration. Yvonne got the bad news of the concentration level from the computer in the plant control room. Immediately she called the plant's dye house. "Paul, this is Yvonne, I think we've got a problem. I'm showing an elevated concentration of red dye in the effluent."

"Now wait a minute, Yvonne, all my instruments show that everything's fine. Are you sure?" came the reply.

"Well, I'm on my way to check it out right now, but I needed to let you know first. My printout shows that we exceeded plant standards about an hour ago." Yvonne answered. "So it might be a good idea to start troubleshooting." Yvonne hung up the phone and drove out to the plant's effluent-monitoring station by the river, checked the instrumentation and confirmed that the control room readout was correct. Then she took her own sample of effluent, and even before it was analyzed, she knew that the instruments weren't lying. There in the test tube was the evidence: water colored pale pink from the dyeing operations.

In the preceding scenario, Yvonne tells Paul, "I'm showing an elevated concentration of red dye in the effluent." **Concentration** refers to the number of molecules or atoms of a substance relative to the space that the substance occupies. In the case of solutions, concentration refers to the amount of solute contained in a unit volume of solution. A solution with a lot of solute is said to be highly concentrated. A solution with a small amount of solute is said to be less highly concentrated, or more **diluted**.

As the concentration of a substance changes, properties of the solution also change. In the preceding scenario, Yvonne monitored the plant effluent through instrumentation. The amount of light absorbed by the solution, as reported by her instruments, told her the concentration of the dye in the effluent. When she saw the pink color of the effluent, she could confirm that the concentration was higher in the effluent than it should have been. The property of the solution—in this case, color, had changed as the concentration of the solute had changed. Later on in this subunit, we will talk about other properties of solutions that change according to the concentration of solutes.

Concentration is expressed in many different ways. It can be expressed as percent by weight, percent by volume, grams per milliliter, moles per liter, or equivalents per liter. The units for these expressions are explained in the next few pages. We will examine them in three groups: molar concentration, normal concentration and percent composition.

Molar Concentration

Molar concentration is the most common concentration used by chemists. It is defined as the number of moles per liter of solution. One mole is by definition 6.02×10^{23} molecules. But don't panic—you don't have to count the molecules. In order to get one mole of a compound, simply weigh in grams one formula weight. Recall from Subunit 1 that the formula weight is the sum of the atomic weights of the elements in the molecular formula. To get those atomic weights, you will need to use the periodic table (Figure 3-7).

Suppose you needed to make a one molar solution of sodium bicarbonate ($NaHCO_3$).

- First, you need the formula weight of sodium bicarbonate, which you can find by consulting the periodic table and adding the atomic weights of each element in the molecular formula $NaHCO_3$, $23 + 1 + 12 + (16 \times 3) = 84$ grams per mole. This tells you that it takes 84 grams of $NaHCO_3$ to make a one molar solution of sodium bicarbonate.

- You then weigh 84 grams of sodium bicarbonate. Dissolve it in a small quantity of water.

- Add enough water to bring the total volume to one liter.

What if you wanted a 0.25 molar solution (expressed as 0.25 M)? If you want any concentration other than 1 M, you simply multiply the desired concentration by the molecular formula weight. For example, to make a 0.25 M $NaHCO_3$ solution, multiply 0.25 mole times 84 grams per mole to get 21 grams. Then dissolve 21 grams of $NaHCO_3$ in a small amount of water and add enough water to bring the volume to one liter of solution.

Suppose you need only a small amount of a sodium bicarbonate solution instead of a full liter. If you want only 250 milliliters of the 0.25 M $NaHCO_3$ solution, you will multiply the 21 grams of $NaHCO_3$ by 250 milliliters and divide that by 1000 milliliters per liter. In doing this, you are finding the weight of the solute that you will need. If you want more than one liter, carry out the same calculation.

Figure 3-7
Periodic Table

PERIODIC TABLE OF THE ELEMENTS

KEY: Atomic Number → 1; Atomic Weight → 1.01; Symbol of Element → H; Name of Element → Hydrogen

GROUP IA	IIA	IIIA	IVA	VA	VIA	VIIA	VIIIA			IB	IIB	IIIB	IVB	VB	VIB	VIIB	GROUP VIIIB
1 1.01 H Hydrogen																	2 4.01 He Helium
3 6.94 Li Lithium	4 9.01 Be Beryllium											5 10.81 B Boron	6 12.01 C Carbon	7 14.01 N Nitrogen	8 16.00 O Oxygen	9 19.00 F Fluorine	10 20.18 Ne Neon
11 22.99 Na Sodium	12 24.30 Mg Magnesium											13 26.98 Al Aluminum	14 28.09 Si Silicon	15 30.97 P Phosphorus	16 32.06 S Sulfur	17 35.45 Cl Chlorine	18 39.95 Ar Argon
19 39.10 K Potassium	20 40.08 Ca Calcium	21 44.96 Sc Scandium	22 47.90 Ti Titanium	23 50.94 V Vanadium	24 52.00 Cr Chromium	25 54.94 Mn Manganese	26 55.85 Fe Iron	27 58.93 Co Cobalt	28 58.70 Ni Nickel	29 63.55 Cu Copper	30 65.38 Zn Zinc	31 69.72 Ga Gallium	32 72.59 Ge Germanium	33 74.92 As Arsenic	34 78.96 Se Selenium	35 79.90 Br Bromine	36 83.80 Kr Krypton
37 85.47 Rb Rubidium	38 87.62 Sr Strontium	39 88.91 Y Yttrium	40 91.22 Zr Zirconium	41 92.91 Nb Niobium	42 95.94 Mo Molybdenum	43 (98) Tc Technetium	44 101.07 Ru Ruthenium	45 102.91 Rh Rhodium	46 106.4 Pd Palladium	47 107.87 Ag Silver	48 112.41 Cd Cadmium	49 114.82 In Indium	50 118.69 Sn Tin	51 121.75 Sb Antimony	52 127.60 Te Tellurium	53 126.90 I Iodine	54 131.30 Xe Xenon
55 132.91 Cs Cesium	56 137.33 Ba Barium	57-71 Below	72 178.49 Hf Hafnium	73 180.95 Ta Tantalum	74 183.85 W Tungsten	75 186.21 Re Rhenium	76 190.2 Os Osmium	77 192.22 Ir Iridium	78 195.09 Pt Platinum	79 196.97 Au Gold	80 200.59 Hg Mercury	81 204.37 Tl Thallium	82 207.2 Pb Lead	83 208.98 Bi Bismuth	84 (209) Po Polonium	85 (210) At Astatine	86 (222) Rn Radon
87 (223) Fr Francium	88 (226) Ra Radium	89-103 Below	104 (261)	105 (262)	106 (263)	107 (262)	108 (265)	109 (266)									

The A & B subgroup designations used with elements in rows 4, 5, 6, and 7, are recommended by the International Union of Pure and Applied Chemistry. Some authors and organizations use the opposite convention for these subgroups.

57 138.91 La Lanthanum	58 140.12 Ce Cesium	59 140.91 Pr Praseodymium	60 144.24 Nd Neodymium	61 (145) Pm Promethium	62 150.35 Sm Samarium	63 151.96 Eu Europium	64 157.25 Gd Gadolinium	65 158.93 Tb Terbium	66 162.50 Dy Dysprosium	67 164.93 Ho Holmium	68 167.26 Er Erbium	69 168.93 Tm Thulium	70 173.04 Yb Ytterbium	71 174.97 Lu Lutetium
89 (227) Ac Actinium	90 232.04 Th Thorium	91 (231) Pa Protactinium	92 238.03 U Uranium	93 (237) Np Neptunium	94 (244) Pu Plutonium	95 (243) Am Americium	96 (247) Cm Curium	97 (247) Bk Berkelium	98 (251) Cf Californium	99 (252) Es Einsteinium	100 (257) Fm Fermium	101 (258) Md Mendelevium	102 (259) No Nobelium	103 (260) Lr Lawrencium

Activity 3-9

- Write in your ABC notebook a description of how you would make 1500 ml of a 0.35 M NaCl solution.

  Note: NaCl is an empirical formula, but the salt does not exist as a molecule except in the vapor phase at high temperatures. Under the extreme conditions of vapor phases, the NaCl molecule has a molecular formula of NaCl. Therefore, when making molar solutions of any salt of a strong acid and a strong base, use the empirical formula for the salt.

Activity 3-10

A mole of something is its molecular mass (formula weight) in grams. So when we talk about a mole of water or anything else, we are referring to its molecular mass expressed in grams.

- Find the mass of the following examples
  - 2 moles of KCl
  - 1.5 moles of $AgNO_3$
  - 4 moles of $CaCO_3$
  - 2.5 moles of H_2SO_4
  - 5 moles of NH_4OH

JOB PROFILE: PHARMACEUTICAL TECHNICIAN

Mali D. is a technician in a pharmaceutical manufacturing company. The company makes many therapeutic products, but Mali works in an area that manufactures a blood-chemistry analyzer. The analyzer is capable of running many different tests on blood samples, such as cholesterol level, different hormone levels, blood sugar, triglycerides, and other components of blood. Before each blood analyzer leaves the plant, even before it goes to the quality-control department, it has to undergo trial runs.

Mali's job is to make up what the technicians call "chemistries," which are solutions that mimic real blood samples. These solutions are able to verify that the readout that the machine gives is correct, because the content of each solution is already known.

To make up the solutions, Mali follows precisely the "recipes" provided by the senior scientist. Some parts of the job are automated, and she oversees the instrumentation and equipment for these operations. "I had done this kind of thing in my college chemistry lab a few times," she says, "but my experience was very limited. I'll never forget how scared I was at the job interview. They were asking me if I knew how to make up molar solutions, normal solutions, how to do titrations, all kinds of things I had learned and forgotten! They taught me to do a lot of it on the job, but they wanted somebody who would have enough knowledge to be easy to train."

Normal Concentration

The **normality** of a solution is defined as the number of equivalents of solute per liter of solution. In other words, a normal solution is measured in the units known as equivalents per liter.

What is an equivalent? An **equivalent** is the weight of solute that will supply one mole of reacting material in a solution. In the case of a type of reaction known as an acid-base reaction, the reacting material would be ions—one mole of hydrogen ions (H^+) or hydroxide ions (OH^-). In reactions known as redox reactions (reduction-oxidation reactions), the reacting material would be electrons—one mole of electrons that are accepted or donated.

This concentration unit—the equivalent—is useful in a laboratory procedure called titration. In a **titration**, a volume of a sample solution is measured. Then a measured amount of a solution that reacts with the sample (for example, a base is added to an acid) is added a small amount at a time until the reaction between the two solutions is completed.

How is the equivalent weight determined? The equivalent weight is found by dividing the molecular weight of the solute by the number of hydrogen ions, hydroxide ions, electrons accepted, or electrons donated—depending on the type of solution.

Let's consider the preparation of one liter of a 0.05 N $Ca(OH)_2$ solution.

- The molecular weight of $Ca(OH)_2$ is $40 + 16 + 16 + 1 + 1 = 74$ grams per mole.
- Each molecule will supply 2 hydroxide ions (OH^-), so the equivalent weight of $Ca(OH)_2$ is 74 grams (the molecular

weight of the solute) divided by 2 (the number of hydroxide ions that are donated), or 37 grams per equivalent.

- For one liter of a 0.05 N solution of $Ca(OH)_2$, 0.05 equivalent is needed. We then multiply 37 grams per equivalent times 0.05 equivalent to get 1.85 grams of $Ca(OH)_2$ needed to make one liter of solution.

Activity 3-11

- Write in your ABC notebook a description of how you would make 4000 ml of a 0.03 N $Ca(OH)_2$ solution.
- Compare your description with that of another student in the class. If they are very different, have your teacher check them both to find out why.

Percent Composition

Percent composition is the most common way of expressing concentration outside the chemistry lab. Percent composition can be expressed in two ways: percent by weight and percent by volume. Percent by weight is used when the solute is a solid. Percent by volume is used when the solute is a liquid.

Percent by Weight

Percent by weight is expressed as the mass in grams of solute per 100 grams of solution. For example a 5% sugar solution contains 5 grams of sugar in 100 grams of solution.

Percent by weight solutions are easy to make. If we want 250 grams of a 5% by weight solution of NaCl in water, we take the following steps:

- Find 5% of 250 grams. This is $250 \times 0.05 = 12.5$ grams.
- Weigh a container that will hold the solution. Then, add weight on the balance to equal 12.5 grams added to the weight of the container.
- Add NaCl to the container on the balance until the scale is balanced.
- Now add weight on the balance to equal 250 grams added to the weight of the container.

- Add water to the container of NaCl until the scale is balanced again.
- Stir the solution thoroughly until all of the NaCl is dissolved. Then transfer the solution to another container for storage.

Activity 3-12

- Write in your ABC notebook a description of how you would make 500 grams of a 10% by weight sugar solution.

Percent by Volume

Percent by volume is used for liquid solutes. Percent by volume is usually expressed as the volume in milliliters of a liquid solute in 100 milliliters of solution. For example, in a 10% by volume solution of acetic acid, there are 10 milliliters of acetic acid in 100 milliliters of solution.

In the alcoholic beverage industry, the amount of alcohol in a given liquor, beer or wine is expressed as "proof," which is twice the actual percent by volume. Therefore, a liquor that is labeled "90 proof" contains 45% alcohol and approximately 55% water and other substances.

When you add ethylene glycol, or antifreeze, to the cooling system of a car, you are mixing a solution of water and antifreeze. The usual percent by volume is 50% antifreeze to 50% water. In a small car, in which the cooling system holds 8 quarts, 4 quarts of antifreeze would be added.

Germicidal Math

Shirley M. is a nurse who is currently working for a home nursing care agency. This week she is taking care of a baby who is home from the hospital after having a tracheostomy, a surgery in which a small hole was made in his windpipe and a plastic tube inserted through the front of the neck to allow him to breathe through the windpipe. The baby was born with a very small upper airway, and he will have a tracheostomy until his airway grows or he is old enough for further surgeries to help open it up.

An important part of Shirley's job is the cleaning and disinfecting of equipment that is required for his care: a suction machine, a fine-mist humidifier, his "trach" tubes, catheters, sterile water jars, etc. All of the equipment that does not actually touch the baby is cleaned daily in a germicide solution. The germicide is very powerful and must be diluted to be used safely.

Shirley reads the instructions that someone—presumably another nurse—has handwritten on the germicide container, "Mix 0.2% by volume for cleaning all respiratory equipment."

"Well, why didn't they just give the measurements?" she asks in an exasperated tone. "But okay, I can figure this out. I know that 0.2% by volume is 0.002 × 1000 milliliters of water, so I need 2 milliliters of germicide to mix up 1000 milliliters of solution. 1000 milliliters is one liter, and I need at least three liters of solution to soak all this tubing in. So that would be 6 milliliters of germicide. Ah, and here's a container to mix it in," she says as she rummages through the supply cabinet. "But just to be sure, I'll call the case manager and make sure that my proportions are correct."

Activity 3-13

- Write in your ABC notebook a description of how you would make 6 liters of a 5% by volume germicidal solution.

Dilution

You have read that concentration refers to the amount of solute contained in a unit volume of solution. A solution with a lot of solute is said to be highly concentrated. A solution with a small amount of solute is said to be less highly concentrated, or more diluted. Sometimes it is desirable to dilute a solution by adding more solvent to it.

If water is the solvent, dilution to a desired concentration can easily be made for any of the concentration units discussed in the preceding pages. If water is not the solvent, this method can still be used with all of the units discussed except percent by weight.

Calculating Dilution to a Desired Concentration

The product of the concentration and the volume gives the amount of solute. To dilute a solution to either a new concentration at an unknown volume or a new volume at an unknown concentration, simply use Equation 3-1:

$$C_1 \times V_1 = C_2 \times V_2 \qquad \textbf{Equation 3-1}$$

where: C_1 = the original concentration

V_1 = the original volume

C_2 = the new concentration

V_2 = the new volume

If you are diluting to a known volume at an unknown concentration, Equation 3-1 can be rearranged to give Equation 3-2:

$$C_2 = C_1 \times \frac{V_1}{V_2} \qquad \textbf{Equation 3-2}$$

If you are diluting to a known concentration at an unknown volume, Equation 3-1 can be rearranged to give Equation 3-3:

$$V_2 = V_1 \times \frac{C_1}{C_2} \qquad \textbf{Equation 3-3}$$

These equations will work as well for molar or normal solutions as they do for percentage solutions.

Activity 3-14

- In your ABC notebook, write a description, complete with calculations, of how you would dilute the following solutions:
  - A dilution of 1 liter of 70% alcohol to 3 liters
  - A dilution of 1 liter of 70% alcohol to 20% dilution
  - A dilution of 2 liters of 1.2 N HCl to a 0.5 N HCl solution

Colligative Properties

Earlier you read the story of how Yvonne, the textile plant technician, noted that the textile plant effluent was pink. The pink color confirmed to her that the amount of solute (red dye) had exceeded acceptable limits and had changed a property of the effluent solution (in this case, its color). The change in concentration (in this case, an increase) had changed the property of the effluent solution.

Another example of how the property of a solution can be changed by the addition of a solute is the use of antifreeze in automobile cooling systems. The addition of ethylene glycol to the water in the car's cooling system changes an important property of the water solution: its freezing point.

In the case of antifreeze, somehow the addition of a solute has lowered the freezing point of the water solution. We also know that salt water freezes at a lower temperature than fresh water. What could the solute ethylene glycol and the solute salt have in common that lowers the freezing point of water?

The answer to this question is surprising. Solutes lower the freezing point of water, not because of their chemical identities, but because of the number of particles present in the solution. Solutes also lower the vapor pressure of a liquid solvent, meaning that the solutions will stay in the liquid phase at higher temperatures if they contain solutes.

Properties such as vapor pressure and freezing point that are determined by the number of solute particles in a solution rather than by the chemical properties of the solute are called **colligative properties**.

In some industrial situations in which it is desirable to keep water in a liquid state, it is useful to be able to change the concentration of liquid solutions in order to change their colligative properties.

Activity 3-15

- Visit the site of your water habitat study.
- Take a reading of the air temperature. Suspend the thermometer about 1 foot above the surface of the water for 5 minutes. Read and record the temperature of the air.
- Take a reading of the water temperature. Suspend the thermometer in the water at a depth of about 1 foot for 5 minutes. Read and record the temperature of the air.
- Take a reading of the light penetration. Use a Secchi disk provided by your teacher. The Secchi disk should be on a line attached to a long pole. Attach the fishing float 1 foot above the Secchi disk. Lower the Secchi disk into the water until the float is in the water. Repeat this procedure, moving the float up one foot each time, until you cannot see the Secchi disk. Measure the distance between the Secchi disk and the float. Record this distance as the distance of light penetration.

Looking Back

Water is withdrawn from surface and groundwater sources for domestic, agricultural and industrial use. Worldwide, agriculture takes the lion's share, 70%, and industry takes about 23%, with domestic use taking the remaining 7%. In the U.S. and other more industrialized countries, industry use generally exceeds agricultural use. Agricultural use of water is primarily for irrigation. Industries use water as a solvent, a coolant, a transporter of materials, a lubricant, among other uses.

One of the most important uses of water is as a solvent. All solvents follow the rule of "like dissolves like." Water is a polar solvent and, like other polar solvents, will dissolve polar solutes. Nonpolar solvents dissolve nonpolar solutes. Soaps, which have one polar end and one nonpolar end, aid water in dissolving nonpolar solutes by forming spheres in which the nonpolar solute can be held.

Concentration refers to the amount of solute contained in a unit volume of solution. Concentration can be expressed as percent by composition (weight or volume), moles per liter, or equivalents per liter. Molar concentration is the most common expression of concentration by chemists. Normal concentration, expressed in equivalents, is useful when a solution is being mixed a small amount at a time until a given reaction between two solutions is completed. This process is called titration. Percent by weight and percent by volume are used to express concentration for many solutions used outside the laboratory.

Sometimes it is desirable to dilute a solution by adding more solvent to it. Dilution can be calculated easily by using a simple equation: $C_1 \times V_1 = C_2 \times V_2$.

Vapor pressure and freezing point of water and other solvents can be lowered by the addition of solutes. The change in properties that occurs with the addition of solutes is the result of the number of solute particles in the solution, rather than as a result of the chemical properties of the solutes.

Further Discussion

- Solution chemistry is an important part of the science of nutrition because the presence of many nutrients is more easily detected in the blood than in body cells and tissues. Investigate, through library sources or with a serologist, how nutrients are detected in the blood.
- Chromatography is a method used by chemists and other scientists to separate and analyze the components of a solution. Research the process in the library and find out where it is used in industry.

Activities by Occupational Area

General

Antifreeze Concentrations

- Contact a mechanic and ask him or her to demonstrate how the antifreeze concentration in a car is tested and how he or she would report this finding to the service manager. Report your findings to the class.

Agriculture and Agribusiness

Pesticide or Fertilizer Solutions

- Contact a farm supply store and find out how a particular pesticide or fertilizer should be mixed with water before spraying. For the smallest quantity of chemical available, calculate how much water must be added to apply it and how much acreage of crop could be treated.

Health Occupations

Solutions from the Pharmacist

- Interview a pharmacist to find out what expression of concentration he or she uses most frequently (on the job). Ask about routine calculations involving concentration, and present them to the class.

Home Economics

Lemonade for the Masses

- Find a lemonade or limeade recipe in a cookbook (or from someone you know).
- Express the amount of pure lemon or lime juice that is dissolved into the water as a percent by volume.
- Express the amount of sugar that is dissolved into the lime- or lemon-and-water solution as a percent by weight.
- Using the percent by composition expressions above, create a new recipe for making 25 gallons of lemonade or limeade.

Industrial Technology

Industrial User Water Return Rate

- Contact the water-quality agency that oversees water quality for your city or region. Find out what percent of water withdrawals from surface water and groundwater in your region is made by industrial users.
- Find out what businesses or manufacturers are the top five water users in your area.
- Contact the person in charge of water use at these industries to find out what percent of the water used must be treated before it can be reused.
- Share your finding with the class.

LAB 2

WHEN SHOULD I SWEETEN MY TEA?

PREVIEW

Introduction

"Mmmmmmm, that's good tea! How does your mother make it, Susan?" says Raymond.

"She has a secret. She dissolves the sugar right after she has brewed it, before it has a chance to cool off," Susan replies.

"Why does that make a difference?"

"She says the sugar dissolves better in the hot tea."

"Well, whatever she does really works. This tea is great!"

Purpose

In this lab, you will study the effect of temperature on the solubility of a commonly used solid—table sugar or sucrose.

Lab Objectives

When you've finished this lab, you will be able to—

- Determine the relative amount of sugar that will dissolve in hot water and in cold water.

Lab Skills

You will use these skills to complete this lab—

- Measure the mass of a substance with a balance.
- Measure the temperature of a substance with a thermometer.

Materials and Equipment Needed

triple-beam balance

hot plate

spatula

glass stirring rods, 2

thermometers, 2

1000-ml beaker

250-ml beaker, 2

100-ml graduated cylinder

two small plastic bowls

sucrose, 400 g

ice, 1 pound

distilled water, 200 ml

safety goggles

LAB PROCEDURE

Method

Put on your lab apron and goggles.

1. Measure and pour into each of the 250-ml beakers 100 ml of distilled water. Label the beakers hot and cold.
2. Place the hot beaker on the hot plate and place a thermometer into the hot beaker. Set the hot-plate control on high and watch the temperature of the water. Decrease the hot-plate control as the temperature approaches 85°C. Increase or decrease the hot-plate control to keep the temperature between 85°C and 90°C.
3. Fill the 1000-ml beaker with ice and water.
4. Place the cold beaker in the ice-water bath and place the thermometer into the cold beaker.
5. Weigh a 200-gram sample of sugar (sucrose) into each of the two plastic bowls.
6. When the temperature of the cold beaker reaches less than 5°C, record the temperature of the cold beaker in the Data Table.
7. Pour one of the 200-gram samples into the cold beaker.
8. Stir the solution with the glass stirring rod for 5 minutes or until all of the sucrose dissolves.

9. Describe what you observe in the Data Table.
10. After the temperature of the hot beaker has reached 85°C, record the temperature of the hot beaker in the Data Table.

11. Add the remaining 200-gram sample of sugar to the hot beaker.

12. Stir the solution with the glass stirring rod for 5 minutes or until all of the sucrose dissolves.
13. Describe what you observe in the Data Table.

Data Table

Beaker	Temperature	Observations
Cold		
Hot		

Calculations

There are no calculations for this lab.

Cleanup Instructions

- Pour the solutions into the sink.
- Wash the glassware and put it in its proper place.

WRAP-UP

Conclusions

1. Which beaker dissolved the sugar more easily?
2. How does the result of this lab compare to what you know about the solubility of gases like carbon dioxide in cold and hot water?

Challenge Question and Extension

3. Describe an experiment that would measure the mass of sugar dissolved in the water.

LAB 3

HOW DOES ANTIFREEZE WORK
PART 1: FREEZING POINT DEPRESSION

PREVIEW

Introduction

Dear Louis:

Thanks for the great birthday card with the picture of the lemur eating birthday cake. I'm not sure what you were trying to tell me, but don't worry, I can take a joke.

You'll never guess what happened. For my birthday, Mom and Dad bought me a car! I couldn't believe it! Before your eyes get too big, though, I should tell you, this is not a status automobile. It's a 1977 Toyota Corolla with 135,000 miles on it. But still, I have wheels! I was so happy I drove it almost all day on Saturday. On Monday after school, Mom drove me over to see our mechanic and said, "Charles, I want you to teach Max how to take care of this car." So after talking it over for a while, they arranged for him to give me a car maintainance lesson every week, in exchange for my being his "gofer," which means, as Charles puts it, "if I need something, you go for it," mostly down to the parts store and back. So one afternoon a week after school, I have a job and I get about a twenty minute "lesson" a week.

The first one was a long lecture about keeping the oil changed. Charles told me all the horror stories he could think of about teenagers with new $50,000 cars with ruined engines from not adding oil and not changing oil. Then he finally showed me how to change the oil.

The next lesson was about antifreeze. Sometimes I think Charles thinks he's Socrates (you know, the Greek guy who taught his students by asking them questions). He starts out, "Max, what is the freezing point of water?" Luckily I remembered it's 0°C or 32°F. "Right," he says, "And in the winter, it gets much colder than that around here. What do you think would happen to your engine if the water in your cooling system froze?" I guessed that it would be like the time our pipes froze and broke. "Right again," he says. (Lots of flair, this guy has.) Anyway, he goes on to tell me about how antifreeze works by lowering the freezing point of water.

Well, Louis, I'm telling you all this because I know you're really into chemistry and so maybe you'll understand it. All this antifreeze action seems to come down to something called colligative properties, and I hope you'll explain it to me the next time you come to visit. And I'll give you a ride in my car! More later—

Your cousin,

Maxine

Purpose

In this lab, you will determine the mixture of antifreeze that provides the greatest protection from freezing.

Lab Objective

When you've finished this lab, you will be able to—

- Choose the antifreeze mixture that provides the most protection from freezing and explain why you chose it.

Lab Skills

You will use these skills to complete this lab—

- Safely handle material from a –86°C temperature bath (dry ice/acetone).
- Determine the relative melting temperatures of a series of mixtures by measuring the time required for each sample to melt in a constant temperature bath.

Materials and Equipment Needed

- 700 g antifreeze
- six 4-inch test tubes
- one 600-ml beaker
- paper towels
- dry ice, 5 lb
- acetone
- timer
- wax pencil
- heat resistant gloves
- six 1-pint bottles
- two droppers
- one liter distilled water
- ice, 5 lb
- 1-liter Dewar flask, one per class
- test-tube holder
- triple-beam balance
- funnel

LAB PROCEDURE

Pre-Lab Discussion

Some of the temperatures in this lab are too cold to measure with the thermometers in your lab. The temperature of the dry ice/acetone mixture is –86°C or -123°F. These temperatures are necessary to freeze the samples and some of the samples may not freeze even at these temperatures.

Instead of measuring the temperatures, you will determine the time required for the mixture to melt as it warms from a temperature of – 86°C to 0°C. The warming does not occur in a linear manner, but along a curve called an exponential. The characteristic temperature versus time curve for a sample warmed from –86°C to 0°C is—

Typical Warming Curve

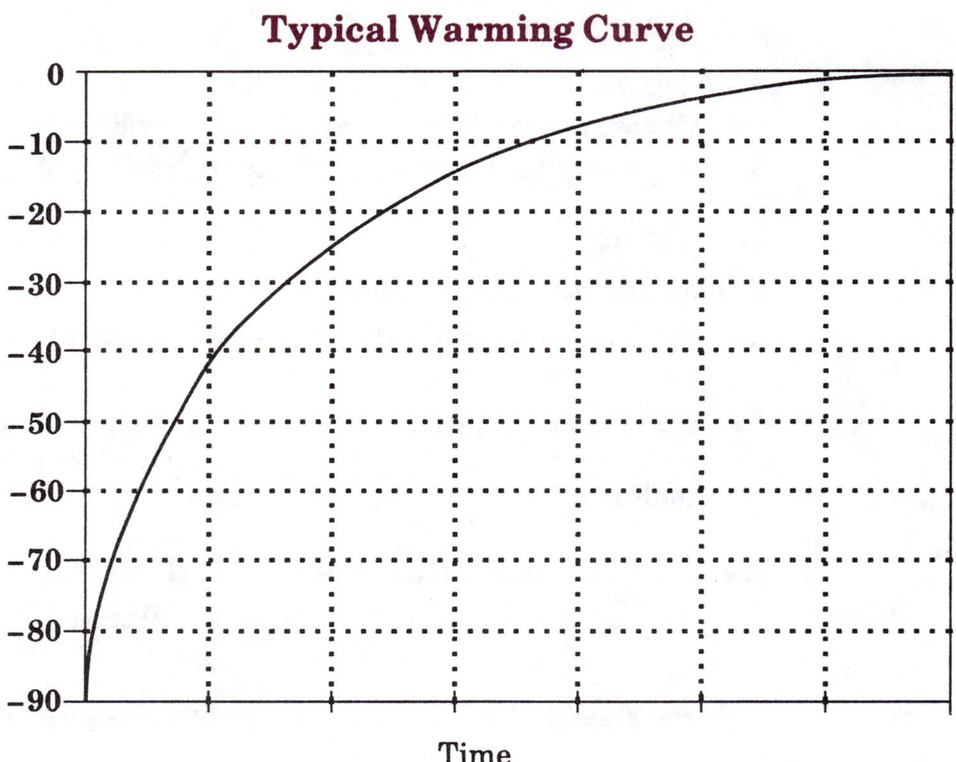

The actual time for the sample to reach the 0°C temperature depends on the mass and thermal properties of the sample. If you have similar quantities in similar test tubes, the warming curves should be similar. If the warming curves are similar, the time required for the sample to melt gives a measure of the relative order of the melting points. The mixture with the highest melting point will take the longest time to melt and the sample with the lowest melting point will take the shortest time to melt.

> **Safety Precautions**
>
> - Be careful not to spill the dry ice/acetone mixture on your skin or clothing. You can get severe frostbite from the cold mixture.

Method

Put on your lab apron and goggles now.

1. Label the 1-pint bottles—0%, 10%, 25%, 50%, 75%, and 100%.
2. Weigh the 600-ml beaker on the triple beam balance.
3. Add 25 grams more weight to the beaker weight on the balance and slowly add antifreeze until balance is achieved. As you get close to the balanced condition, add the antifreeze a drop at a time with a dropper.
4. Add 225 grams more weight to the beaker and antifreeze weight and slowly add distilled water until balance is achieved. As you get close to the balanced condition, add the distilled water one drop at a time with a dropper.
5. Use the funnel and pour this solution into the bottle labeled 10%.
6. Wash and dry the beaker.
7. Repeat Steps 2 through 6 for the following weights and percentage solutions—

0%	no antifreeze	250 g water
25%	62.5 g antifreeze	187.5 g water
50%	125 g antifreeze	125 g water
75%	187.5 g antifreeze	62.5 g water
100%	250 g antifreeze	no water

8. Pour about 300 ml of tap water into the 600-ml beaker. Add ice to bring the total volume in the beaker to about 450 ml.
9. Pour the 100% solution into a 4-inch test tube to a level of about 2 inches.

10. Wearing heat resistant gloves, use the test-tube holder to immerse the test tube in the dry ice/acetone slush for 2 minutes.

11. At the same time, you move the frozen sample from the dry ice/acetone slush to the beaker of ice and water. Your lab partner should start the timer. DO NOT LET THE LEVEL OF THE WATER GET ABOVE THE TOP OF THE TEST TUBE.
12. Observe the sample as it melts. Record the time when the melting completes as melting time in the Data Table.
13. Repeat Steps 9 through 13 for each of the other solutions.

Data Table

Solution	Melting time
0% antifreeze	
10% antifreeze	
25% antifreeze	
50% antifreeze	
75% antifreeze	
100%antifreeze	

Cleanup Instructions

- Wash the glassware and return it to its proper place.
- Pour the solutions back into the appropriate 1-pint bottles and save the solutions for Lab 3.

Calculation

1. Draw a graph of the concentration versus the melting time. Label the x-axis antifreeze concentration and the y-axis melting time.

WRAP-UP

Conclusions

1. Is the graph of your data a straight line? Should it be?
2. Discuss what concentration of antifreeze would provide the most protection from freezing? Would this be 100% antifreeze? Why?

Challenge Question and Extension

3. When the solutions inside a cell freeze, the solution often expands, rupturing the cell membrane. What kind of plant breeding program would develop plants that are less vulnerable to this kind of freeze damage?

LAB 4

HOW DOES ANTIFREEZE WORK PART 2: BOILING POINT ELEVATION

PREVIEW

Introduction

Dear Louis,

Congratulations on your moving up to first chair in the trombone section of the school band. It's great that you get into the games free, too.

My main extracurricular activity this semester is still my car maintainance lessons with Charles. I think he might be dragging out my lessons because he likes having my help around the garage, but I don't really mind. For one thing, every time he sends me down to the parts store, I run into all these guys from school.

Thanks for the info on colligative properties. I was wondering how antifreeze could make the freezing point lower and make the boiling point higher, but when you consider that it's a matter of the number of particles added to water, it makes more sense. I asked Charles what you asked me about how hot most cars get in 100 degree weather like you have down there in Texas in the summer. He said that on the open highway, where there's a lot of air circulating, the engine temperature can get up to 220°F, and in a Houston traffic jam, it could easily go up to 240°F or 250°F. The "opening point" (I'm learning all this car talk—that's the temperature at which the car starts off) can be 192°F to 198°F. In old cars, it's lower, but that's another story—how cars have changed and why—that Charles loves to tell. Anyway, he said that if you wanted to protect a car from 100 degree weather, you would do it by using a mix of at least 50% antifreeze and 50% water (percent by volume), and that you might even go up to 60% antifreeze. Then he showed me how the cooling system works, and that was pretty interesting.

How did your algebra test turn out? I'm doing okay in algebra this year—even after a rough start. Bye now.

Your cousin

Maxine

Purpose

In this lab, you will determine the mixture of antifreeze that provides the greatest protection from boiling in the summer.

Lab Objective

When you've finished this lab, you will be able to—

- Determine which antifreeze solution gives the radiator coolant with the highest boiling point for summer use.

Lab Skill

You will use this skill to complete this lab—

- Measure the boiling point of a liquid sample.

Materials and Equipment Needed

solutions from Lab 2

one 500-ml Erlenmeyer flasks

hot plate

ring stand with 2 clamps

thermometer

wax pencil

funnel

boiling chips

heat-resistant gloves

LAB PROCEDURE

Pre-Lab Discussion

In the summer, an added burden is often placed on an automobile's cooling system. Air conditioning causes the engine to work harder, producing more heat. In heavy, stop-and-go traffic, less air moves through the radiator to carry the heat away. These conditions can cause the coolant in the radiator to boil, building up pressure to the point that the pressure must be released by the radiator cap. When the radiator cap releases the pressure, the radiator loses some of the coolant. The loss of coolant only makes the problem worse.

To lessen the problem, antifreeze is used in the summer to increase the boiling point of the coolant. With the proper mixture of antifreeze, the boiling point of the coolant can be increased to 150°C or more. The increase in the boiling point of the coolant keeps the coolant from boiling and building up pressure that must be released. The higher boiling point of the coolant makes the cooling system of a car work more efficiently in the summer.

Safety Precautions

- Be careful when removing the hot flask from the hot plate. Spilling the hot liquid on clothing or skin can cause painful burns.

Method

Put on your lab apron and goggles now.

1. Obtain an antifreeze solution from your teacher. Record the percentage of antifreeze in the solution. Each lab station will run a boiling point determination on distilled water and one antifreeze solution.
2. Set up the apparatus as shown in Figure L3-1.

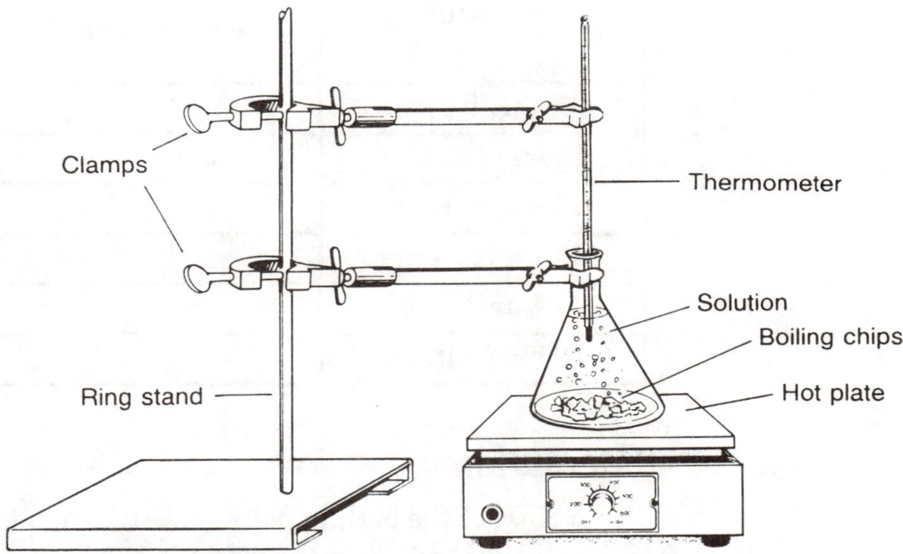

Figure L3-1 Set up of boiling point determination apparatus

3. Pour 200 ml of distilled water into the flask, put 4 boiling chips in the flask, and place the thermometer in the water.
4. Turn on the hot plate.

5. After the water boils for 3 minutes, read the thermometer. Record this value in the Data Table as the boiling point of 0% antifreeze.

6. Turn off the hotplate.
7. Wearing heat resistant gloves, use tongs to pour the water in the flask down the sink. Dry the flask.

9. Repeat steps 3 through 6 for your assigned antifreeze solution.
10. Allow the antifreeze solution to cool. Then pout it back into its storage bottle.
11. Write the value for the boiling point of your assigned antifreeze solution on the board.
12. Copy the Data Table into your lab notebook. Then record the boiling points for the other antifreeze solutions in the Data Table.
13. Save the solutions for Lab 4.

Data Table

Solution	Boiling temperature	Boiling point elevation
0% antifreeze		
10% antifreeze		
25% antifreeze		
50% antifreeze		
75% antifreeze		
100% antifreeze		

Calculations

1. Subtract the boiling point of water from the boiling point of each solution and enter the value in the Data Table as the boiling point elevation.
2. Draw a graph of the concentration versus the boiling point elevation. Label the x-axis antifreeze concentration and the y-axis boiling point elevation.

Cleanup Instructions

- Throw the used boiling chips in the trash.
- Wash the glassware and return it to its proper location.

WRAP-UP

Conclusions

1. Is the graph of your data a straight line? Should it be?
2. Discuss what concentration of antifreeze would provide the most protection from boiling? Would this be 100% antifreeze? Why?

LAB 5

HOW IS DENSITY MEASURED?

PREVIEW

Introduction

Dear Louis,

Mom just got off the phone with Aunt Leah, and she said that your leg is in a cast! Something about falling off the bleachers during a game, but Mom didn't get the story straight. (She never gets the details.) What happened? I hope you can still play this fall with the band. Anyway, write me soon and tell me about it.

My last lesson with Charles was on Tuesday, and boy, did I get a big surprise. At the end of the lesson, he said, "Well, Max, I got you a little graduation present for finishing all these auto maintainance lessons," and he handed me a box with a tire gauge and a hydrometer in it! Then he said, "I think you'll need these if you decide to accept my job offer." Then he offered me a job working at the garage, mostly out front pumping gas, but hey, it's going to be real money!

The hydrometer is cool. Do you know what one is? It's used to check the antifreeze in a car cooling system. This one looks like a turkey baster. Charles explained to me that a hydrometer works by measuring specific gravity. When antifreeze is added to the water, it changes its specific gravity (that's the ratio of the density of a substance to the density of water). You can tell if you've got enough antifreeze or too much by checking the specific gravity.

My hydrometer doesn't have a reading of specific gravity, though. It has all these little colored balls. Each ball has a different density, and they float or not according to the density of the liquid in the hydrometer. Anyway, you have to see it to really understand it.

Isn't it great about the job? When are you going to come visit? You can come and watch me check the oil in people's cars.

Your cousin,

Maxine

Purpose

In this lab, you will find the relationship between density and concentration.

Lab Objectives

When you've finished this lab, you will be able to—

- Measure the density of a liquid.
- Relate density or specific gravity to concentration.

Lab Skills

You will use these skills to complete this lab—

- Use a hydrometer to measure specific gravity.
- Use a graduated cylinder and triple-beam balance to measure density of a liquid.

Materials and Equipment Needed

antifreeze solutions from Lab 3

one 100-ml graduated cylinder

one triple-beam balance

six droppers

hydrometer, 1 per class

LAB PROCEDURE

Pre-Lab Discussion

For solutes that have a density less than 1 g/cm^3 or greater than 1 g/cm^3, but not equal to 1 g/cm^3, density is a good indicator of concentration. If the density is less than 1 g/cm^3, the less solute in a solution, and the less the density will be. If the density is greater than 1 g/cm^3, the more solute in the solution, and the greater the density will be. This gives a convenient way to determine the concentration of a solution. The density or specific gravity (density of substance divided by the density of water) is easy to measure. For antifreeze, a common hydrometer has four plastic balls. The number of balls that float gives an indication of the freezing point of the solution (related to the concentration).

Method

Put on your lab apron and goggles.

1. Weigh a clean, dry 100-ml graduated cylinder.

2. Using a dropper for the last portion, add 100 ml of distilled water to the graduated cylinder.
3. Weigh the filled graduated cylinder. Record the weight in the Data Table for 0% antifreeze.
4. Return the solution to its storage bottle.
5. Clean and dry the graduated cylinder.
6. Repeat Steps 1 through 4 for each antifreeze solution.
7. Use the hydrometer to determine the specific gravity of distilled water and each antifreeze solution that falls within the range of the hydrometer. Record the measured specific gravity in the Data Table.

Data Table

Solution	Weight	Density	Measured Specific Gravity	Calculated Specific Gravity
0% antifreeze				
10% antifreeze				
25% antifreeze				
50% antifreeze				
75% antifreeze				
100% antifreeze				

Calculations

1. Divide the weight of each solution by 100.
2. Record the answer for each solution as the density in the Data Table.
3. Divide the density of each solution by the density of water. Record this value as the calculated specific gravity in the Data Table.
4. Graph concentration versus density.
5. Graph density versus specific gravity.

Cleanup Instructions

- Wash the glassware and return it to its proper location.
- Give the antifreeze solutions to your teacher for disposal.

WRAP-UP

Conclusions

1. How does the density compare to the values of specific gravity for each solution?
2. How does the measured specific gravity compare to the calculated specific gravity?
3. How does the density vary with concentration?
4. Can you use density to determine concentration? Explain.

SUBUNIT 4

What Are Acids and Bases and How Are They Used in Solutions?

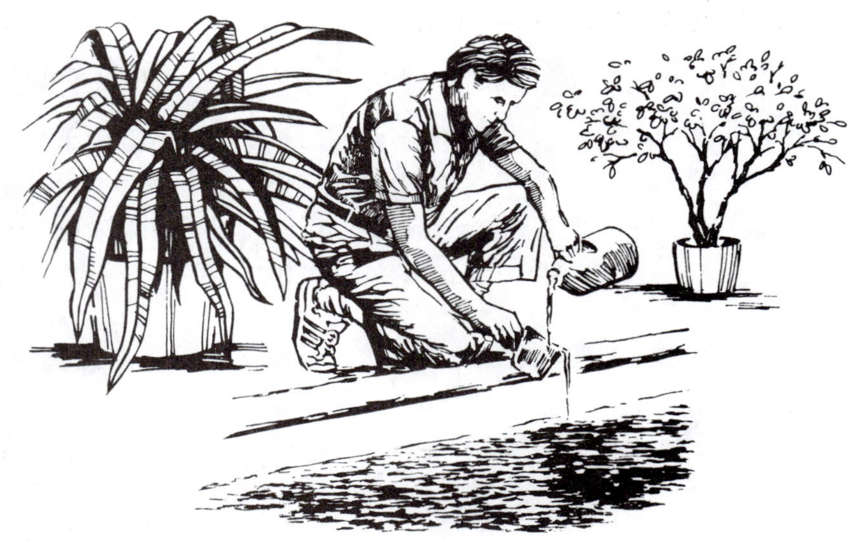

THINK ABOUT IT

- The man in the picture above is adding a small amount of muriatic acid (a solution of hydrochloric acid) to lower the pH of a swimming pool. Imagine that this is a pool where you usually go swimming. Which of the following best reflects your reaction to the use of acid to clean the pool?

  a. You would never swim in a pool that had any type of acid put into it for any reason.

  b. You assume that adding acid to the pool water will irritate your eyes and skin.

  c. You assume that acids are okay as long as they are mixed with enough water to be weak.

  d. You don't care how the pool is cleaned as long as it doesn't have green scum in it.

  e. You'd like some assurance that this guy knows what he's doing. Does he know the chemistry involved? Does he know how to follow directions?

SUBUNIT OBJECTIVES

After you complete this subunit, you will be able to —

1. Identify at least three commonly used acids and three commonly used bases.
2. Contrast the ionization of pure water with the ionization that occurs in an acidic or basic solution.
3. Calculate the concentration of hydroxide ions, given the concentration of hydrogen ions, and vice versa.
4. Explain the relationship between the molar concentration of hydrogen ions and the pH scale.
5. Predict how a hazardous acid spill might be neutralized and list the factors of the spill that would have to be taken into consideration.
6. Explain what is meant by the use of the words strong and weak in relation to acids and bases.
7. Predict what kind of substance might act as a buffer for a strong acid and in what kind of situation buffering might be useful.

What Are Acids and Bases?

Peeling an Onion

Ms. Li sees Veronica and Leroy in the hall at lunchtime. "How's the research going?" she asks them. "Have you two figured out the who, when, where and how of water use yet?"

"Oh, don't ask," says Leroy, groaning. "This research project is like peeling an onion. Every layer has another layer under it."

"I can believe it," Ms. Li responds. "Water chemistry—that's really what you're dealing with—is a complex subject."

"We're doing okay," Veronica says. "We've got a little of the who and the where and at least a piece of the how. I mean, we know some industries that use a lot of water. We don't know that much about how different water uses affect water

quality. But we know about how water dissolves materials and how important that is in the way it's used."

"Good start, I'd say," says Ms. Li.

Leroy goes on, "Yeah, but you know, Ms. Li, I thought that by now we'd be closer to an answer to the problem of Hondo Springs."

"What kind of answer do you mean?" asks Ms. Li.

I guess I thought that we would find a list somewhere—good industries and bad industries. These guys use it up; those guys put something really bad in it, like some evil acid, or something. But it's not that clear," he finishes up.

"No," says Ms. Li, "in this case, it really isn't. And it's especially hard to sort out unless you understand the chemistry. In fact, when I think about what you just said about evil acid, it occurs to me that you might need to do a little research on acids and bases."

"Peeling the onion again?" asks Leroy. "And what are bases. I guess you don't mean first base or home base, do you?"

* * *

Later on in the cafeteria, Veronica says, "I can't believe we have to do more research now on acids and bases. If you had just kept your 'evil acid' theory to yourself! Anyway, all acids aren't bad, you know. In fact, you're eating two acids right now."

"What do you mean?" Leroy asks, big-eyed.

"Acetic acid in the vinegar in your salad dressing," Veronica says, "and citric acid in the lemon in your iced tea!"

Acids have a bad reputation. People often think of acids as "evil" chemicals, the kind that burn holes through metal and pollute **groundwater**. In some cases, this is true, but there are acids that are not corrosive or polluting. Solutions made from acids and from another group of chemicals called bases are useful in many different ways. Let's look again at the way that acids and bases were defined in Subunit 1.

Acids are substances that, when they are mixed with water, react to form **hydronium ions:** $\mathbf{H_30^+}$. (You may remember from other units that **ions** are particles that carry a positive or negative charge. An ion is formed when an atom or a group of atoms gains or loses electrons.)

Many foods contain acids. Oranges and lemons contain citric acid. Souring milk contains lactic acid. Fermented cider forms acetic acid. Many acids are used in industry. One of the most important is sulfuric acid. It is used in petroleum refining, steel processing, and fertilizer production. Phosphoric acid and nitric acid are two other important industrial chemicals; they are used primarily in making fertilizers. Some commonly used acids are shown in Figure 4-1.

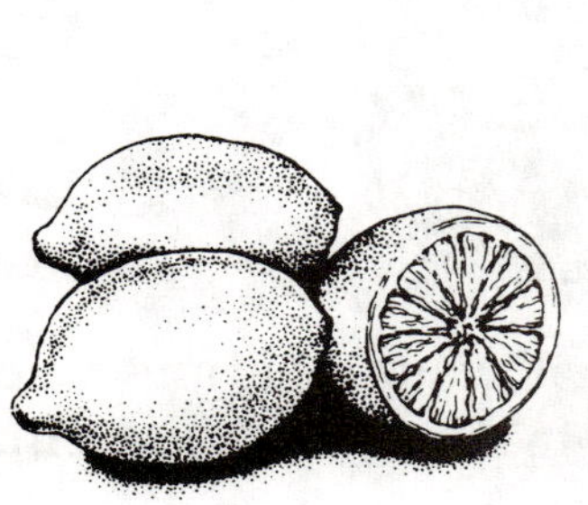

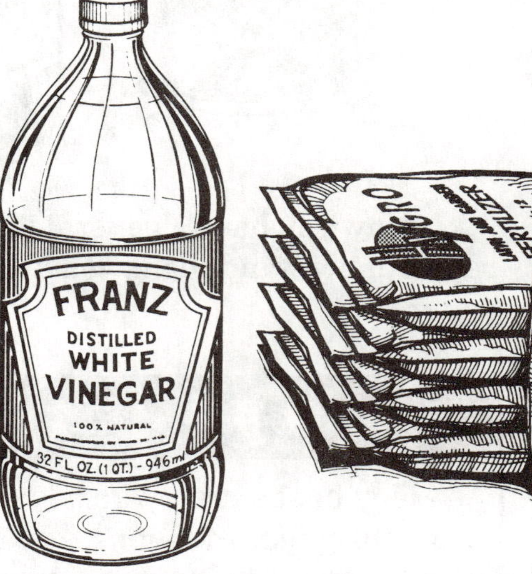

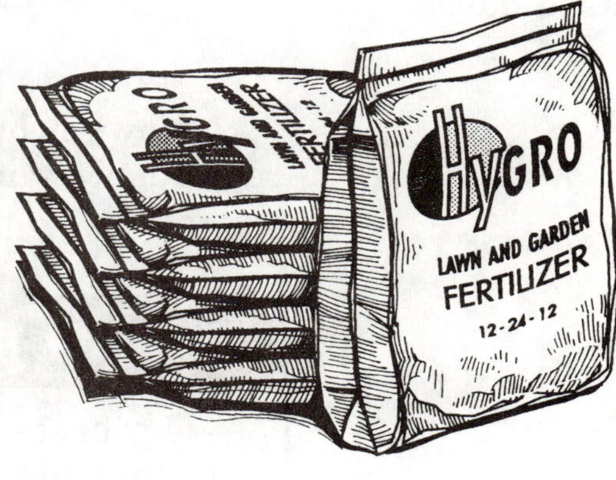

Figure 4-1
Some commonly used acids or products made with acids

Activity 4-1

- Do an inventory of acids found in food products. Check product labels at your local supermarket.
- Answer the following questions: What acids are frequently found in food products? In what types of foods are acids most frequently listed as an ingredient? What types of food processing, if any, are associated with the use of acids in foods?

Bases are substances that form **hydroxide ions, OH^-**, when they are mixed with water. Bases are found in nature and are also commercially prepared. Several basic solutions are found in most people's homes. For example, household ammonia is a basic solution used for cleaning floors and other surfaces. Milk of magnesia is found in many home medicine cabinets and is used as a stomach antacid to treat indigestion. Some commonly used bases are shown in Figure 4-2.

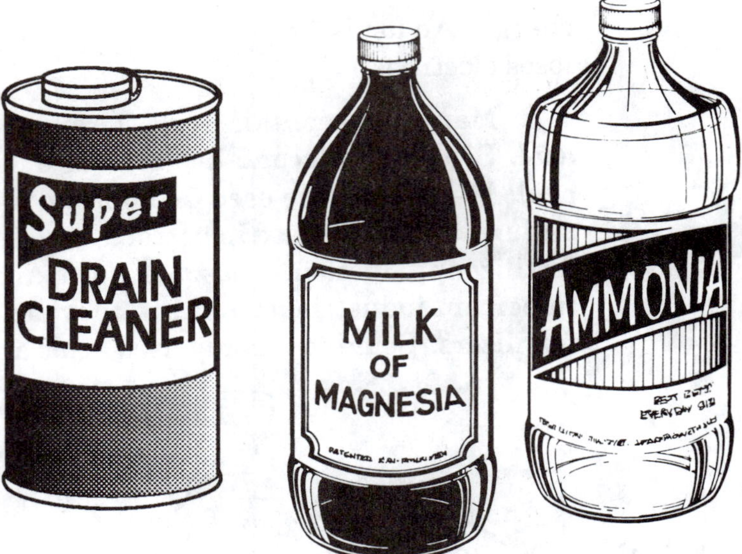

Figure 4-2
Some commonly used bases

Now you have a general idea of what acids and bases are, but to really understand them, you need to know about the ionization of water.

Activity 4-2

Many bases are hydroxides; that is, they are compounds that contain hydroxide ions.

- Survey the antacid counter of a pharmacy or grocery store. Read the labels of antacid tablets to find out if they contain hydroxides.
- Record the name of the hydroxide and the product name.
- Answer the following questions: What are the main ingredients (listed among the first) of these products? How does one antacid differ from another, as far as you can tell from the label?

How Does Water Ionize?

You read in Subunit 3 that the polarity of water molecules causes them to cling to each other to some extent. The negative end of one water molecule is attracted to the positive end of another water molecule, and so on. These attractions are called hydrogen bonds.

Hydrogen bonding is partly responsible for the ionization of water. Every now and then, the collisions between water molecules are so energetic that one of the molecules breaks apart—ionizes. The ionization reaction is represented as—

$2H_2O$	$\rightarrow$	H_3O^+	+	OH^-
water		hydronium ion		hydroxide ion

Equation 4-1

This reaction is called the **ionization of water**, or sometimes, the **self-ionization of water**. Figure 4-3 shows a diagram of hydronium and hydroxide ions.

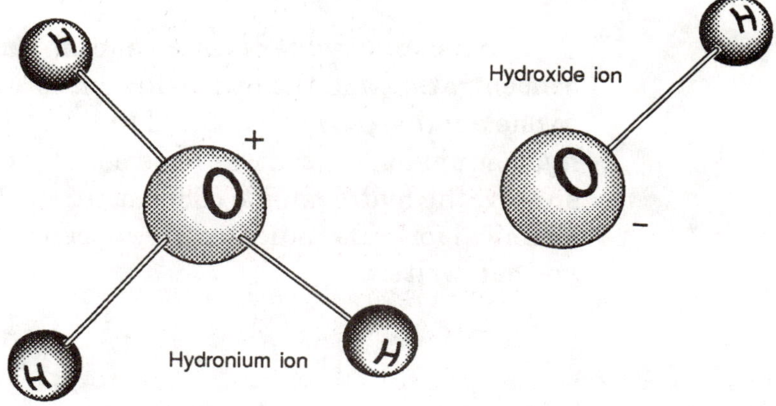

Figure 4-3 Hydronium and hydroxide ions

How does hydrogen bonding aid the process of ionization? The attraction of the partially postive hydrogen and the partially negative oxygen weakens the bond between the hydrogen and oxygen. The weakened water bond may be broken with relative ease because the positive charge of the hydrogen ion is stabilized by the partially negative oxygen atom in the hydrogen bond.

When ionization occurs, the ions are immediately surrounded by water molecules. The hydroxide (OH^-) ion is surrounded by water molecules with the partially positive hydrogens pointing to the negative oxygen of the OH ion to stabilize the charge. The positive charge on the remaining hydrogen atom (remaining from the molecule that broke apart) is stabilized by distributing it to the other two hydrogens on the hydrogen-bonded water molecule, forming what is called a hydronium ion (H_3O^+). The hydronium ion is surrounded by water molecules pointing their oxygen atoms (with their partially negative charges) toward the positive hydrogen atoms.

In pure water, ionization takes place to a very limited extent. In distilled water at 25°C, only one in every 556,000,000 molecules present (1.0×10^{-7} moles per liter) ionizes.

The ionization reaction of water reaches an equilibrium. **Chemical equilibrium** is the condition in a chemical reaction in which the reactants are converting to products at the same rate that the products are converting back to reactants. Therefore, the ionization of water shown in Figure 4-1 can be written with two arrows, like this:

$$\underset{\text{water}}{2H_2O} \rightleftharpoons \underset{\text{hydronium ion}}{H_3O^+} + \underset{\text{hydroxide ion}}{OH^-}$$

Equation 4-2

When pure water is at an equilibrium, the hydronium ion concentration and the hydroxide ion concentration are always equal to one another, so each is equal to 1.0×10^{-7} moles per liter. The hydronium ion concentration is usually written as $[H^+]$ and called, simply, the hydrogen ion concentration. Using brackets around the chemical formula indicates the concentration in moles per liter. Thus you can write:

$$[H^+] = 1.0 \times 10^{-7}$$

Equation 4-3

$$[OH^-] = 1.0 \times 10^{-7}$$

Equation 4-4

The two equations show what was said earlier: the concentrations of hydrogen ions and hydroxide ions in pure water are equal to one another. Pure water, then, is said to be neutral. Any water solution in which the $[H^+]$ and the $[OH^-]$ are equal to 1.0×10^{-7} is called a **neutral solution**.

Activity 4-3

For many industries, it is necessary to use pure water. The diagram below represents a common method of purifying water. In fact, the deionized water you may be using in your lab may have been produced by this method, called ion exchange.

Column 1 in the diagram contains a resin embedded with ionizable hydrogens. A cation (which can generally be represented as B^+) is any atom or group of atoms with a positive charge. When a solution containing cations passes through column 1, the B^+ cations exchange with the ionizable hydrogens and remain in the column.

Column 2 contains a resin embedded with hydroxide ions. An anion (which can be represented as A^-) is any atom or group of atoms with a negative charge. When a solution containing an anion passes through Column 2, the A^- anions exchange with the hydroxide ions and remain in the column. So, when water containing a salt (B^+A^-) passes through the ion-exchange system, cations of the salt are exchanged for the hydrogen ions in the resin in Column 1 and anions of the salt are exchanged for the hydroxide ions in the resin in Column 2.

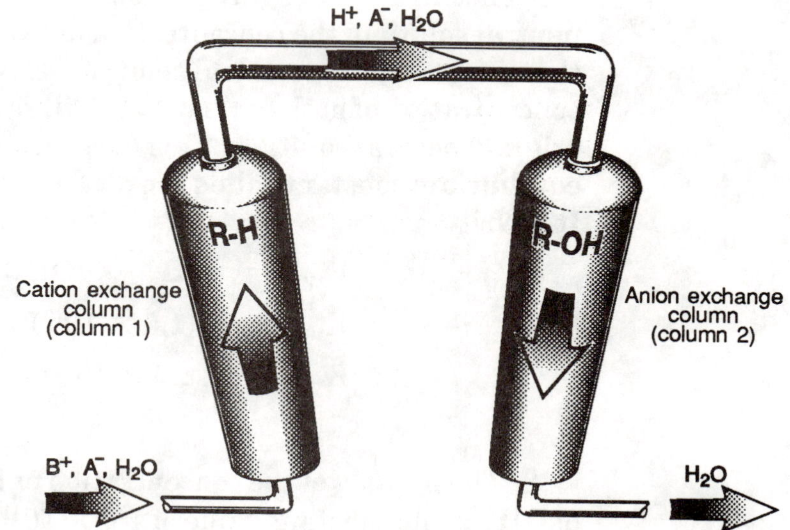

- Explain how passing salt water through the ion-exchange system above could produce pure water (pH = 7).

How Does the Ratio of Hydrogen Ions Change in Water Solutions?

The equilibrium that is set up in pure water is not unique. Other water solutions can also reach equilibrium in the ionization reaction. Some water solutions have more hydrogen ions than hydroxide ions. Other water solutions have more hydroxide ions than hydrogen ions. But they can still reach equilibrium. How is this possible?

Equilibrium Constant

The answer is that Le Chatelier's principle is at work. Remember that Le Chatelier's principle states that a system at equilibrium that is disturbed will move to reestablish equilibrium. Therefore, if one type of ion (either hydrogen ions or hydroxide ions) is added to a neutral water solution, then the system will shift to decrease the other type of ion.

Here's how Le Chatelier's principle works in this situation. If H^+ ions are added to a neutral solution, OH^- ions combine quickly with the excess H_3O^+ ions, forming new water molecules. This lowers the concentration of both the H^+ ions and the OH^- ions until a new equilibrium is established. When the new equilibrium is established, the concentration of hydrogen ions will be higher than in the original neutral solution; the concentration of hydroxide ions will be lower than in the original neutral solution. However, the product of the concentration of both types of ions will remain the same as in the original neutral solution. This idea is expressed by a special kind of equilibrium constant called the dissociation constant of water, or K_W. It is written:

$$K_W = [H^+] \times [OH^-]$$
$$K_W = (1.0 \times 10^{-7}) \times (1.0 \times 10^{-7})$$
$$K_W = 1.0 \times 10^{-14}$$

Equation 4-5

The *product* of the concentration of H_3O^+ and the concentration of OH^- is the constant value of 1.0×10^{-14} for water solutions at 25°C. Therefore, if you know the concentration of one type of ion, you can always find the concentration of the other.

Activity 4-4

You will need to use the equilibrium constant equation to find the following:

- Find the $[OH^-]$ of a solution with a $[H^+] = 1.0 \times 10^{-6}$.
- Find the $[H^+]$ of a solution with a $[OH^-] = 1.0 \times 10^{-6}$.

Acidic and Basic Solutions

Acid and basic solutions can be defined in relation to their hydrogen ion and hydroxide ion concentrations. However, before we go on to definitions, let's look at an industry in which acid solutions are produced.

Tour of a Fertilizer Plant

Owen S. is a lab technician for a chemical company; he works in a division that makes fertilizer. He has worked for the company a long time, so he's a naturally good person to give tours, which he does once a week.

The plant where Owen works is part of a large complex. In one area, sulfuric acid is made. Sulfuric acid is then combined with phosphates to make phosphoric acid, which is used to make fertilizer.

Owen explains to those of us on the tour, "My job is in the middle of the process, you could say. Fertilizer is made up mainly of sulfuric acid and phosphate. I used to work at the sulfuric acid plant. Even that part isn't simple. It's a three-part process. First they burn sulfur with oxygen to make sulfur dioxide. Then they put the sulfur dioxide through a converter, where it's combined with oxygen to make sulfur trioxide. Finally sulfur trioxide is mixed with water to make sulfuric acid."

He goes on, "Phosphate rock is brought in from a neighboring state. The rock is mixed with water to make a slurry, so it can be transported through the pipeline. When it gets here, the water is separated off and stored for later use. The thickened slurry that's left is fed into the phosphoric acid plant.

"The main reaction in a phosphoric acid plant," Owen explains, "is the reaction between tricalcium phosphate and sulfuric acid to give soluble phosphoric acid and insoluble calcium sulfate, better known as gypsum." He shows us the main reaction on a blackboard in the plant control room, but explains that it actually takes place in two steps:

$Ca_3(PO_4)_2$	+	$3H_2SO_4$	+	$6H_20$	$\rightarrow$	$3CaSO_4.2H_2O$	+	$2H_3PO_4$
tricalcium phosphate		sulfuric acid		water		gypsum		phosphoric acid

"But you can see this isn't like baking a cake," Owen explains. "We don't just put the reactants in a big mixing bowl. We put them into an isothermal reactor—a kind of big pressure chamber. We are standing in the reactor control room." Owen shows us the pressure, temperature and

vacuum readings on the control panel. He explains, "The reaction takes place under controlled pressure and temperature conditions. Temperature probes at the top and bottom of the reactor monitor internal temperatures in the reactor."

Owen takes us into a small laboratory not far from the reactor control room. "This is my area," he says. "The amount of sulfuric acid that needs to be mixed with the phosphate rock varies with the quality of the rock. We test the rock right here in this lab and report our findings to the operations manager in the control room.

"When the phosphoric acid is made, it has to be purified in clarifiers; then it goes into large storage ponds inside the plant." Owen shows us how the acid is eventually used to make a compound called "calcium superphosphate" that is used for the fertilizer.

At the end of the tour, Owen promises us, "Next time you look at a bag of fertilizer and you see 'phosphates' in the list of ingredients, you won't take it for granted."

When acids and bases are added to water, they cause the solution to have an increase in hydrogen ions or hydroxide ions. Let's look again at the definitions of acid and base that were given earlier in the subunit. Now that you have read about the ionization of water, these definitions should make more sense.

Acids are substances that, when they are mixed with water, form hydronium ions. (Remember that hydronium ions are usually written as H^+ and called hydrogen ions.) In acidic solutions, there are more hydrogen ions $[H^+]$ than hydroxide ions $[OH^-]$. Another way to express this is to say that acidic solutions have a hydrogen ion concentration that is greater than 1.0×10^{-7}. The more acidic the solution, the closer the hydrogen ion concentration gets to 1.0×10^{0}.

Bases are substances that, when they are mixed with water, form hydroxide ions. In basic solutions, there are more hydroxide ions than hydrogen ions. Therefore, basic solutions have a hydrogen ion concentration that is less than 1.0×10^{-7}. The more basic the solution, the closer the hydrogen ion concentration gets to 1.0×10^{-14}. Basic solutions are also called **alkaline** solutions.

There is another way to think about and to define what is going on when acids and bases react. That is, we can consider that a proton is being donated or accepted. An acid—with its hydrogen ions—can be defined as a substance that donates protons to a solution. A base—

because it produces hydroxide ions—can be defined as a substance that accepts a proton from an acid.

This way of defining acids and bases—as proton donors and proton acceptors—was developed independently by two scientists named Brønsted and Lowery. So you will sometimes hear the terms "Brønsted-Lowery base" or "Brønsted-Lowery acid."

What Is pH?

Activity 4-5

- Visit the site of your habitat study.
- Carefully fill a sample bottle with water from the sampling site. Be sure not to bubble the air out of the sample bottle. Instead, hold the mouth of the bottle at the water surface and let the water run into the bottle gently. When the bottle is filled, screw the cap tightly on the bottle.
- When you return to the lab, measure the pH of the water with pH paper or a pH meter. Record the pH value of the water from the sampling site.

Leroy Says No to Logarithms

Leroy and Veronica are going over what they've learned about acids and bases with Ms. Li. "The thing that really gets me," says Veronica, "is why we have to use this clumsy way of telling the molar concentration of hydrogen ions and hydroxide ions. Do you ever think scientists just like to make things more complicated so they use scientific notation?"

Leroy breaks in, "Maybe you think it would be better if you had to write out all those zeros? That would be a lot more trouble."

"He's right," Ms. Li says. "But you have a point, Veronica. Writing out the molar concentration of acids and bases is cumbersome. That's why we use the pH scale."

"The pH scale? I remember we measured pH at Hondo Springs, but I didn't really know what it meant," says Veronica.

"pH is a measure of how acidic or basic—alkaline—a solution is," explains Ms. Li.

"I remember now," says Leroy. "The scale goes from 0-14; 0 is acid city and 14 is, like, the most milk-of-magnesia you can get."

"Right," says Ms. Li, "well, more or less. Milk-of-magnesia actually has a pH of around 10, not 14, but you've got the idea; it's alkaline."

"So if you can use a number from 0 to 14, why bother with this molar concentration stuff?" asks Veronica.

"Because that's where we get the pH scale," says Ms. Li, "from the molar concentration of hydrogen ions and hydroxide ions. pH is the negative logarithm of the hydrogen-ion concentration."

"Stop, stop right now, Ms. Li," Leroy holds up his hand. "We went to city council hearings. We went to Hondo Springs to test the water and survey the life forms. We have been to the Chamber of Commerce to get lists of industries. Now we've been studying solutions and acids and bases. But we are not going to study logar-, logar-, heck, I can't even pronounce it. We are not going to study those things so we can figure out what to do with Hondo Springs! Right, Veronica? Right?"

"Uh, well, uh," stutters Veronica.

"Don't panic, Leroy," says Ms. Li. "You don't have to study logarithms right now—although I'm sure you wouldn't find them too difficult. A logarithm is a mathematical expression that can be found easily with a calculator."

Activity 4-6

Use a calculator with a log function on it to carry out these operations.

- Enter the number 1.0×10^{-7}.
- Press the log function key.
- Press the key to change signs.

After carrying out these operations, you should have 7 showing in the calculator display. The number is the pH of a solution with a hydrogen ion concentration of 1.0×10^{-7} moles per liter. The definition of the pH is the negative logarithm of the hydrogen ion concentration.

The **pH scale** is a system that indicates the acidity or alkalinity of a solution. The pH scale ranges from 0 to 14. The numbers correspond to the hydrogen-ion concentration of the solution (Figure 4-4); they are the **negative logarithm** of the hydrogen-ion concentration. A **logarithm** is the exponent that indicates the power to which a number has been raised to produce a given number.

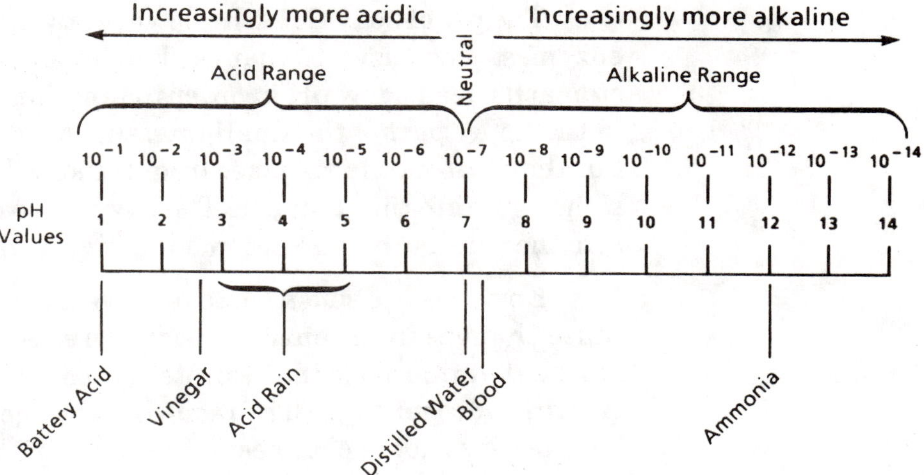

Figure 4-4
pH scale

Activity 4-7

pH can be tested using a paper permeated with litmus, a dye that changes color according to exposure to acidic or alkaline solutions.

- Use litmus paper to test the foods you identified as containing acids in Activity 4-1.
- Test other household solutions, from the medicine cabinet, the cleaning supplies, and the refrigerator.
- Make a chart in your ABC notebook or with a group of classmates, to indicate which substances are acidic and which are alkaline.

You may be wondering: what about the molar concentration of hydroxide ions? Are they indicated by the pH scale? The negative logarithm of the molar hydroxide-ion concentration can be calculated to arrive at **pOH**. A neutral solution would have a pOH of 7. A solution with a pOH less than 7.0 is basic, greater than 7.0 is acidic. However, we don't use a pOH scale because we don't need one. If we know the pH, we can always calculate the pOH by using the equation for the equilibrium constant for solutions.

The pH of a solution is a critical indicator of how the solution will function. Especially in living systems, pH must stay within a certain range in order for life to be maintained. We will examine some of the ways that pH affects living systems.

Enzyme Activity and pH

The pH of body fluids has a very strong effect on the activity of enzymes. The enzymes that work to break down the food in our stomachs need a low pH in order to function. The enzymes that work in the upper part of the small intestine need a higher pH to function. For that reason, the enzymes from the small intestine become inactive if they get into the stomach. The enzymes from the stomach that pass into the small intestine become inactive as the pH increases.

Enzymes are sensitive to pH levels because pH changes actually cause changes in the enzymes' structure. At different pH levels, different amino acids in the protein become ionized. That is, they lose or gain hydrogen ions. The resulting change in the charge of the amino acids causes changes in the shape of the enzyme molecule. When the enzyme changes shape, the molecules it is supposed to break down or put together do not fit the enzyme anymore, so it becomes inactive.

Environmental pH and Acid Rain

Some air pollutants can combine with water in reactions that create acid rain. Two classes of air pollutants that can have such effects are the oxides of sulfur, commonly called SO_x and the oxides of nitrogen, commonly called NO_x. The x in these chemical formulas indicates the presence of more than one oxide. SO_x and NO_x can dissolve in water in the atmosphere in a way that is similar to the reaction in the body between carbon dioxide and water that produces carbonic acid. SO_x and NO_x can produce rain that has a pH less than 5. Rain at or below pH 5 is commonly referred to as **acid rain.**

Acid rain can affect plant growth in two ways: by directly damaging plant leaves or by making the soil so acidic that it interferes with the plant's ability to absorb nutrients. (Some plants grow well in slightly acidic soil, but very acidic soil usually inhibits plant growth.)

Acid rain affects water environments, too. It may damage the aquatic plants upon which fish feed. The water itself may become too acidic to support fish and other aquatic life.

How Do Acids and Bases Neutralize One Another?

JOB PROFILE: Chemist

Rosalinda C. is a chemist in her state's Hazardous Chemical Emergency Response Unit. Her office houses the state's "hot line" for hazardous chemical cleanup. When a chemical spill occurs, Rosalinda is often one of the first to hear about it. If it's a serious spill, she usually calls one of the eighteen state inspectors to go and see about it. She may also consult with the contractor who is cleaning up the spill.

"Often the decision is made to neutralize the spill of an acid or a strong base," Rosalinda explains. "With an acid, for example, lime or soda ash might be used. Lime and soda are both basic substances, so they interact with acids to form water and a salt."

She goes on, "First response has to be based on the specific conditions of a spill. If you spill a water-soluble acid in a river—say, sulfuric acid—there's not a lot you can do. A few years ago, we had just such a spill in this state. Sulfuric acid was spilled into a river. There was an attempt by the company to clean it up by putting lime into the river. But the sulfuric acid had already moved down the river, killing fish for 12 miles. The lime never reacted with the sulfuric acid. Instead, it reacted with the water, which led to more fish kills. That's why we now have a state office like this one.

"We have to be very careful about how we respond to a chemical accident. We have to know where it occurred—on asphalt, cement, soil, or inside a building. We have to know the geology of the spill site. We have to estimate how much of the chemical was spilled, how strong it is, etc.

"Neutralization often makes a spill much easier to handle. Take, for example, an acid spill that has been neutralized by coating the ground where it occurred with lime ash. The lime absorbs the acid, which neutralizes it. The next step usually is to remove the neutralized material and a portion of the soil. We test the removed material and the remaining soil. Then we have to find a proper disposal site for the removed material." Rosalinda has a bachelor's degree in chemistry and about nine years of experience as an industrial chemist.

When an acid and a base combine, they react to form water and a salt. Such a reaction is called an **acid-base neutralization** reaction. When an acidic solution is mixed with a basic solution and they react completely, the resulting mixed solution is **neutral**—neither acidic nor basic. In a neutralization reaction, hydrogen ions (contributed by the acid) combine with hydroxide ions (contributed by the base) to form neutral water. For example, hydrochloric acid reacts with sodium hydroxide to produce water and table salt:

HCl	+	NaOH	→	NaCl	+	H_2O
hydrochloric acid		sodium hydroxide		sodium chloride		water

Equation 4-6

The General Reaction

It is useful to be able to predict how an acid and a base will react. To describe the general reaction of an acid and a base, we will use two terms introduced in Activity 4-3: anion and cation. To review, an **anion** (A^-) is any atom or group of atoms with a negative charge. A **cation** (B^+) is any atom or group of atoms with a positive charge.

In general, an acid, which can be described as HA, will ionize in water to produce a hydrogen ion (H^+) and an anion (A^-). A base, which can be described as BOH, will ionize in water to produce a hydroxide ion (OH^-) and a cation (B^+). The cation is usually a metal ion. The cation (B^+) and the anion (A^-) combine as a result of the neutralization reaction to form a salt. The hydrogen ion and the hydroxide ion combine to form water. The general neutralization equation is shown below:

HA	+	BOH	→	BA	+	H_2O
acid		base		salt		water

Equation 4-7

Activity 4-8

- Identify an industry in your area that uses acids in manufacturing.
- Interview the plant safety officer or other person in charge of safety to find out if the acid is corrosive or otherwise harmful to people or damaging to property. Find out how acid spills are cleaned up and whether they are neutralized using a base.

Salts

A salt is the anion (A^-) from an acid and the cation (B^+) from a base. Table 4-1 lists some common salts, and the anions and cations that form them.

Table 4-1. Some Common Salts and Their Anions and Cations

Chemical name	Chemical formula	Cation	Anion
Sodium chloride	$NaCl$	Na^+	Cl^-
Sodium carbonate	Na_2CO_3	Na^+	CO_3^{--}
Sodium bicarbonate	$NaHCO_3$	Na^+	HCO_3^-
Potassium iodide	KI	K^+	I^-
Calcium carbonate	$CaCO_3$	Ca^{++}	CO_3^{--}
Sodium sulfate	Na_2SO_4	Na^+	SO_4^{--}

Activity 4-9

- Barium sulfate is a salt that is used for diagnostic tests on the gastrointestinal system. Contact a radiologist to find out why and how barium sulfate is used in diagnostic tests.

Strong and Weak Acids and Bases

Sometimes acids and bases are described as strong or weak. You might expect that a strong acid solution is one in which the acid is very concentrated, and that a weak acid is one in which the acid is very diluted. However, that is only partly true.

To say that an acid is strong means that the acid is completely ionized in the water solution. To say that an acid is weak means that only a fraction of its molecules break apart to form ions.

Like acids, bases can be strong or weak. Strong bases are those that dissociate (break apart) completely into metal ions and hydroxide ions in water solutions. Weak bases do not dissociate completely in water solutions.

What Are Buffers and How Do They Resist pH Changes?

The pH of water can be changed very easily. If 0.01 mole of HCl is added to 1 liter of distilled water, the pH will decrease from 7 to 2. If 0.01 mole of NaOH is added to 1 liter of distilled water, the pH will increase from 7 to 12. In each case, the pH changes a full five pH units with the addition of only 0.01 mole of the acid or base. These and similar experiments show us that water does not resist pH change.

A buffer is a solution that resists pH change. When even relatively large amounts of acid or base are added to a buffer solution, the pH remains fairly constant. A buffer may consist of a weak acid and one of its salts or a weak base and one of its salts.

Let's consider a buffer solution containing a weak acid and one of its salts: 0.10 mole of acetic acid (CH_3COOH), a weak acid, and 0.10 mole of sodium acetate (CH_3COONa), a salt of acetic acid, in 1 liter of water. This buffer solution has a pH of slightly less than 5.

The sodium acetate in the buffer solution is ionized as shown below:

$$\underset{\text{sodium acetate}}{CH_3COONa} \rightarrow \underset{\text{acetate ion}}{CH_3COO^-} + \underset{\text{sodium ion}}{Na^+}$$

Equation 4-8

When an acid is added to this buffer solution, the acetate ion, CH_3COO^-, captures the hydrogen ions and makes acetic acid, like this:

CH_3COO^-	+	H^+	→	CH_3COOH
acetate ion		hydrogen ion		acetic acid

Equation 4-9

Because acetic acid does not ionize very completely in water (it is a weak acid), the pH of the solution doesn't change much.

What happens if a base is added to the acetic acid-sodium acetate solution? The base will add hydroxide ions to the solution. The hydrogen ions of the acetic acid will react with the hydroxide ions to produce water, like this:

H^+	+	OH^-	→	+	H_2O
hydrogen ion		hydroxide ion			water

Equation 4-10

The combination of hydrogen ions from the acetic acid with hydroxide ions upsets the balance of hydrogen ions and hydroxide ions, so to maintain equilibrium (remember Le Chatlier's principle), the acetic acid ionizes further.

CH_3COOH	→	CH_3COO^-	+	H^+
acetic acid		acetate ion		hydrogen ion

Equation 4-11

In summary, if an acid is added to a weak-acid-and-salt buffer solution, the hydrogen ions react with the anion from the salt. If a base is added to such a buffer solution, the hydroxide ions react with the hydrogen ions from the ionized acid. Then additional acid ionizes to form new hydrogen ions, thus reestablishing equilibrium in the buffer system.

Many solutions can act as buffers. A mixture of a weak base, like NH_4OH, and a strong acid, like HCl, can form a buffer that is stable in a higher pH range (around pH 9) than the acetic acid-sodium acetate system.

By carefully choosing the weak acid or weak base, you can make a buffer system that can stabilize pH at a desired level. If a weak base and a strong acid are used, the pH usually will be greater than 7. If a weak acid and a strong base are used, the pH usually will be less than 7.

Let's look at two ways that buffering is used, one in the medical setting and one in the environmental field.

Physiological Buffering of Blood

Higher animals have ways of dealing with changes in pH of their body fluids. Mammals have a blood-buffer system. As with the buffer system discussed previously, the term buffer refers to substances that help a solution resist a change in pH. One such pair of substances in blood is the carbonic acid-bicarbonate system.

Here's how the carbonic acid-bicarbonate buffer system defends the blood against a change in pH. In a condition of acidosis, excess hydrogen ions are circulating in the blood. The H^+ ions combine with HCO_3^-, bicarbonate ions (readily available in sodium bicarbonate found in the body) to produce a weak acid.

H^+	+	HCO_3^-	→	H_2CO_3
hydrogen ions		bicarbonate		carbonic acid

Equation 4-12

Now let's take the case of excess base (OH^-) in the blood. In a condition of alkalosis, excess hydroxide ions are circulating in the blood. The hydroxide ions combine with carbonic acid (readily available in the body) to produce water and bicarbonate ions.

OH^-	+	H_2CO_3	→	HCO_3^-	+	H_2O
hydroxide ions		carbonic acid		bicarbonate ions		water

Equation 4-13

The bicarbonate ions produced by this buffering system quickly combine with sodium ions in the body and thus do not upset the pH of the body systems.

Limestone Buffering of Streams and Lakes

Acid rain is a problem in many areas of the country. As you read earlier, oxides of sulfur and nitrogen dissolve in atmospheric water, which falls as acid rain. Acid rain can damage plants, lower the pH of soil and pollute surface waters.

In some areas of the country, acid rain enters surface waters, but it does not have the effect of lowering pH to a significant degree. Why do some areas escape environmental damage to their lakes and streams?

The answer is that some lakes and streams are naturally buffered. They contain large limestone deposits, which are made up primarily of calcium carbonate. Calcium carbonate reacts with the acid through a sequence of reactions:

$$\underset{\text{calcium carbonate}}{CaCO_3} + \underset{\text{water}}{2H_2O} \quad \underset{\text{ion}}{H^+} \rightarrow \underset{\text{calcium hydroxide}}{Ca(OH)_2} + \underset{\text{carbonic acid}}{H_2CO_3}$$

Equation 4-14

The two products on the right side of Equation 4-14 react in water as follows:

$$\underset{\text{carbonic acid}}{H_2CO_3} \rightarrow \underset{\text{water}}{H_2O} + \underset{\text{carbon dioxide}}{CO_2}$$

Equation 4-15

$$\underset{\text{hydrogen ions}}{2H^+} + \underset{\text{calcium hydroxide}}{Ca(OH)_2} \rightarrow \underset{\text{calcium ions}}{Ca^{+2}} + \underset{\text{water}}{2\,H_2O}$$

Equation 4-16

This sequence of reactions causes the pH in lakes and streams that have a limestone geology to remain stable even when acid rain falls into them. Limestone is used to treat some lakes that are not naturally buffered and that have a lowered pH as a result of acid rain.

Activity 4-10

At the beginning of this subunit, you answered a question about the cleaning of a swimming pool. Now that you have more information about acid-base chemistry, you can investigate swimming pool maintainance more thoroughly.

- Call a swimming pool company and arrange to talk to someone who cleans pools or instructs owners on the care and cleaning of pools.
- Find out what chemicals are used in swimming pool maintainance, and with the help of the pool company representative and your teacher, identify the major chemical reactions in pool chemistry.

Looking Back

Acids are substances that, when they are mixed with water, react to form hydronium ions, H_3O^+. Bases are substances that form hydroxide ions, OH^- when they are mixed with water.

Pure water contains some hydronium and hydroxide ions; these are formed when water molecules ionize, or break apart. The molar concentration of hydronium ions is usually written as $[H^+]$ and called, simply, the hydrogen-ion concentration. The hydroxide-ion concentration is written as $[OH^-]$.

The product of the $[H^+]$ and $[OH^-]$ is a constant value, 1.0×10^{-14}, which is called the dissociation constant for water. The equilibrium constant holds true for pure water as well as for acidic and basic solutions. The dissociation constant makes it possible to find the $[H^+]$ if you have the $[OH^-]$, or to find the $[OH^-]$ if you have the $[H^+]$.

The pH scale is a system that indicates the acidity or alkalinity (how basic it is) of a solution. The pH scale ranges from 0-14. The numbers correspond to the hydrogen-ion concentration of the solution.

A neutralization reaction is one in which hydrogen ions contributed by an acid combine with hydroxide ions contributed by a base to form neutral water.

Buffers are solutions that resist pH change. A buffer may consist of a weak acid and one of its salts or a weak base and one of its salts. A buffer works like this: if an acid is added to a weak-acid-and-salt buffer solution, the hydrogen ions react with the anion from the salt. If a base is added to such a buffer solution, the hydroxide ions react with the hydrogen ions from the ionized acid. Then additional acid ionizes to form new hydrogen ions, thus reestablishing equilibrium in the buffer system.

Further Discussion

- The manufacturing of computer chips usually involves the use of acids. Acids are used to etch patterns of circuitry into the silicon wafer that will eventually form the memory chips of the computer. Many different acids have been used in this process. Typically a solution containing phosphoric acid, nitric acid, acetic acid, water and wetting agents is used. Contact a representative from a semiconductor company to visit your class and talk about the use of acids in the chip manufacturing process. Find out what other ways acids are used in the semiconductor industry. What qualities of acids make them suitable for these jobs?

Activities by Occupational Area

General

Hair Products and pH

- Check the product labels of shampoos and other hair products to find any references to pH.
- Share your findings with the class. How can you verify whether there is a scientific basis for a balanced pH in hair-care products?

Agriculture and Agribusiness

Soil Treatment for Alkalinity and Acidity

- Consult your agricultural extension agent to find out whether the soil in your area is primarily alkaline or acidic. Ask for references to growers in the area.
- Interview different growers to find out how they treat the soil for alkalinity or acidity (whichever is appropriate).
- Share your findings as a class and compare and contrast the different methods of soil treatment used by different growers.

Health Occupations

Measurement of Blood pH

- Visit a hospital and talk to a respiratory therapist to find out how blood pH is measured.
- Find out who installs and maintains the equipment used in blood pH measurement.
- Find out what different blood pH readings tell the respiratory therapist about the condition of the patient.

Home Economics

Textile Dyes

- Using product labels to identify and locate companies, write to a company that manufactures textile dyes.
- Ask for information about their products and processes. Inquire specifically about the role of chemical salts in dyeing procedures.
- Share your information with the class.

Industrial Technology

Acids Used in Printing and Printmaking

- Visit a printing company or artist's studio where metal engraving is done. Ask for a demonstration of the process to find out:
    1. What acids are used.
    2. How they are used.
    3. How they are mixed in solution.
- Share your findings with the class.

LAB 6

HOW DOES pH AFFECT HYDROPONIC PLANT GROWTH?

PREVIEW

Introduction

Marie C. is a soil fertility expert for an experiment station associated with a state university agriculture program. Her responsibilities are to study soil characteristics and how these characteristics affect plant growth.

"Soil pH can have a strong effect on the kinds of plants that will grow in a particular soil," says Marie. "Soil pH affects the availability of plant nutrients—low pH can increase the availability of aluminum, iron, manganese, copper, and zinc and decrease the availability of molybdenum, boron, sulfur, calcium, magnesium, potassium, phosphorus, and nitrogen. High soil pH can increase the availability of molybdenum, boron, sulfur, calcium, magnesium, and potassium while it decreases the availability of nitrogen, phosphorus, copper, zinc, iron, manganese, and aluminum."

Marie says that different plants have different requirements for different nutrients and each plant has an optimum pH range where it does the best. If a soil is too acidic for a desired crop, the soil pH can be raised by adding lime to the soil. If the soil is too basic, the soil pH can be lowered by adding sulfur to the soil.

Purpose

In this lab, you will determine the optimum pH range for soybean plants (or other plant assigned by your teacher).

Lab Objective

When you've finished this lab, you will be able to—

- Study the effect of pH on plant growth.

Lab Skills

You will use these skills to complete this lab—

- Measure the pH of a solution
- Adjust the pH of a solution.
- Determine plant growth rates.

Materials and Equipment Needed

- dropper
- nine one-pint bottles
- nine soy bean seedlings
- 0.1 N HCl, 50 ml
- pH paper or pH meter
- wax pencil
- nine Styrofoam or plastic cups
- Perlite or vermiculite, 1 quart
- hydroponic nutrient mixture 4.5 liters
- 0.1 N HaOH, 50 ml
- ruler or meterstick

LAB PROCEDURE

Pre-Lab Discussion

There are some general symptoms of deficiencies of the different plant nutrients. They are listed in Table L5-1.

Table L5-1: Symptoms of Nutrient Deficiency in Plants

Nitrogen	Reduced growth, yellowing of the leaves
Phosphorus	Reduced growth, poor root system, reduced flowering, thin stems, browning or purpling of the leaves
Potassium	Reduced growth, shortened internodes, brown leaf edges, dead spots in the leaf, plants that wilt easily
Calcium	Lack of bud growth, death of root tips, cupping of mature leaves, blossom-end rot, pits on root vegetables
Magnesium	Reduced growth, some yellowing of leaves and leaf veins, cupped leaves, reduced seed production
Sulfur	Yellowing of the entire plant
Iron	Yellowing of leaves and leaf veins in young leaves
Zinc	Yellowing of leaves and leaf veins, reduction in leaf size, short internodes
Molybdenum	Yellowing of leaves and leaf veins in older leaves
Boron	Failure to set seed, death of tip buds
Copper	New growth small and misshapen, wilted
Manganese	Yellowing of leaves and leaf veins, brown spotting

In this lab, you will identify nutrient deficiencies by matching symptoms in Table L5-1 to the appearance of the seedlings growing at different pH levels.

Method

Put on your lab apron and goggles.

1. Divide the 4.5 liters of hydroponic nutrient mixture into nine 500-ml portions.
2. Adjust the pH of the first 500 ml of nutrient mixture portion to a pH of 5 by following the following procedure—
   a. Measure the pH of the solution. If the pH is the desired pH, go to Step F.
   b. If the pH is higher than the desired pH, add one drop of 0.1 N HCl.

   c. If the pH is lower than the desired pH, add one drop of 0.1 N NaOH.
   d. Mix the solution well.
   e. Return to step A and continue until the desired pH is reached.
   f. Pour the solution into a one-pint bottle and label the bottle.
3. Repeat Step 2 with the other eight nutrient mixture solutions adjusting them to pHs of 5.5, 6, 6.5, 7, 7.5, 8, 8.5, and 9 respectively.
4. Choose nine soybean seedlings that are about the same height and plant one in each Styrofoam cup, supporting the seedlings with Perlite.
5. Label each cup with the appropriate pH value from 5 to 9 in 0.5-pH unit increments.
6. Fill each cup with the nutrient mixture with the appropriate pH.
7. Measure the height of each soybean seedling above the top of its Styrofoam cup and record the height in the Data Table.
8. Check the plants each weekday for two weeks.
   - Check the pH of the solution to be sure it has not changed.
   - Add more nutrient mixture of the appropriate pH as it is needed.
   - Measure and record in the Data Table the height of each of the seedlings each day.

Data Table: Daily Height of Seedlings

	Day											
pH	1	2	3	4	5	6	7	8	9	10	11	12
5.0												
5.5												
6.0												
6.5												
7.0												
7.5												
8.0												
8.5												
9.0												

On day 12 write a brief description of each plant.

pH	Appearance of Seedling
5.0	
5.5	
6.0	
6.5	
7.0	

pH	Appearance of Seedling
7.5	
8.0	
8.5	
9.0	

Calculations

1. Calculate the first week's growth rate for each pH by subtracting the day 1 measurement from the day 5 measurement and dividing by 5.
2. Calculate the second week's growth rate for each pH by subtracting the day 8 measurement from the day 12 measurement and dividing by 5.
3. Graph pH versus growth rate for the first week's growth rate and the second week's growth rate.

Cleanup Instructions

- Throw the cups and plants in the trash
- Empty the bottles of nutrient mixture on the school lawn.
- Wash the bottles and return them to their proper location.

WRAP-UP

Conclusions

1. What is the optimum pH range for soybean plants? Explain.
2. What symptoms of nutrient deficiencies can you identify in the plants that appear unhealthy?

3. **Deficiency of which nutrients is consistent with these symptoms?**

Challenge Questions and Extensions

4. **Predict what would happen if the plants that appear unhealthy were put in nutrient solutions that are in the optimum range.**

LAB 7

HOW IS pH LOWERED?

PREVIEW

Introduction

Anita K. is a lifeguard at a large public swimming pool. One of her jobs is to check the pH and chlorine concentration of the water in the pool twice in the morning and twice in the afternoon. She enters the values for the pH into a log. "We use chlorine gas to chlorinate the water at our pool," says Anita, "When chlorine gas dissolves in water, it forms the weak hypochlorous acid (HClO) and hydrochloric acid (HCl). The hydrochloric acid lowers the pH of the water in the pool unless we add a base to neutralize the acid."

The pool where Anita works pumps a sodium hydroxide solution into the water to neutralize the hydrochloric acid. Anita just checked the pH and chlorine levels. The chlorine level is correct, but the pH is 7.8—that is too high. She enters the values in the log and goes to the pump house to adjust the pumping rate on the NaOH.

Purpose

In this lab, you will lower the pH of a distilled water sample by adding 0.1 N HCl to the sample.

Lab Objectives

When you've finished this lab, you will be able to—

- Lower the pH of a solution by adding hydrochloric acid to it.
- Understand the way pH changes as acid is added to a solution.

Lab Skill

You will use this skill to complete this lab—

- Measure pH with a pH meter or pH paper.

Materials and Equipment Needed

250-ml beaker	pH paper or pH meter
0.1 N HCl, 10 ml	dropper
freshly boiled distilled water, 100 ml	

LAB PROCEDURE

Method

Put on your lab apron and goggles.

1. Pour 100 ml of freshly boiled distilled water into a 250-ml beaker.
2. Measure the pH of the water with pH paper or a pH meter. Record the value in the Data Table.
3. Measure the pH of the 0.1 N HCl. Record the value in the Data Table.
4. Add 1 drop of 0.1 N HCl to the water sample. Use the stirring rod to mix the sample. Measure the pH of the mixture and record the value in the Data Table.
5. Repeat Step 4 until 5 drops total have been added.
6. Add 2 drops (total of 7 drops) of 0.1 N HCl to the sample. Use the stirring rod to mix the sample. Measure the pH of the mixture and record the value in the Data Table.
7. Add 3 drops (total of 10 drops) of 0.1 N HCl to the sample. Use the stirring rod to mix the sample. Measure the pH of the mixture and record the value in the Data Table.
8. Add 5 drops of 0.1 N HCl to the sample. Use the stirring rod to mix the sample. Measure the pH and record the value in the Data Table.
9. Repeat Step 8 until the pH change is less than you can detect. On many pH meters, this will be 0.05 pH unit.
10. Add 10 drops of 0.1 N HCl to the sample. Use the stirring rod to mix the sample. Measure the pH and record the value in the Data Table.
11. Repeat Step 10 until the pH change is less than you can detect.
12. Add 20 drops of 0.1 N HCl to the sample. Use the stirring rod to mix the sample. Measure the pH and record the value in the Data Table.
13. Repeat Step 12 until 120 drops total of 0.1 N HCl have been added.

Data Table

Drops Added	pH
0	
1	
2	
3	
4	
5	
7	
10	
15	
120	
0. 1N HCl	

Calculation

1. Graph the volume of 0.1 N HCl added (in drops) versus the pH of the mixture.

Cleanup Instruction

- Wash the glassware and return it to its proper location.

WRAP-UP

Conclusions

1. Do you think you could adjust the pH of a distilled water sample originally at pH of 7 to a pH of 6 using 0.1 N HCl? Explain why.
2. Do you think you could adjust the pH of a distilled water sample originally at pH of 7 to a pH of 3 using 0.01 N HCl? Explain why.
3. In which range would it be most difficult to adjust the pH of a distilled water sample to a specific pH value?

LAB 8

HOW IS pH RAISED?

PREVIEW

Introduction

When Anita decreased the pumping rate of the sodium hydroxide solution to lower the pH of the pool, she decreased it too much. By the next morning, the pH of the pool was down to 6.8—much too low. "It is really hard to set the pump just right," says Anita. "The pH is so sensitive in the range we need that just a small amount has a big effect." She turns to go to the pump house to increase the pumping rate of the sodium hydroxide. "I hope it doesn't bounce back too high this time."

Purpose

In this lab, you will raise the pH of a distilled water sample by adding 0.1 N NaOH to the sample.

Lab Objectives

When you've finished this lab, you will be able to—

- Raise the pH of a solution by adding sodium hydroxide to it.
- Understand the way pH changes as base is added to a solution.

Lab Skill

You will use this skill to complete this lab—

- Measure pH with a pH meter or pH paper.

Materials and Equipment Needed

250-ml beaker

0.1 N NaOH, 10 ml

freshly boiled distilled water, 100 ml

pH paper or pH meter

dropper

LAB PROCEDURE

Method

Put on your lab apron and goggles.

1. Pour 100 ml of freshly boiled distilled water into a 250-ml beaker.
2. Measure the pH of the water with pH paper or a pH meter. Record the value in the Data Table.
3. Measure the pH of the 0.1 N NaOH. Record the value in the Data Table.
4. Add 1 drop of 0.1 N NaOH to the water sample. Use the stirring rod to mix the sample. Measure the pH of the mixture and record the value in the Data Table.
5. Repeat Step 4 until 5 drops total have been added.
6. Add 2 drops (total of 7 drops) of 0.1 N NaOH to the sample. Use the stirring rod to mix the sample. Measure the pH of the mixture and record the value in the Data Table.
7. Add 3 drops (total of 10 drops) of 0.1 N NaOH to the sample. Use the stirring rod to mix the sample. Measure the pH of the mixture and record the value in the Data Table.
8. Add 5 drops of 0.1 N NaOH to the sample. Use the stirring rod to mix the sample. Measure the pH and record the value in the Data Table.
9. Repeat Step 8 until the pH change is less than you can detect. On many pH meters, this will be 0.05 pH unit.
10. Add 10 drops of 0.1 N NaOH to the sample. Use the stirring rod to mix the sample. Measure the pH and record the value in the Data Table.
11. Repeat Step 10 until the pH change is less than you can detect.
12. Add 20 drops of 0.1 N NaOH to the sample. Use the stirring rod to mix the sample. Measure the pH and record the value in the Data Table.
13. Repeat Step 12 until 120 drops total of 0.1 N NaOH have been added.

Data Table

Drops Added	pH
0	
1	
2	
3	
4	
5	
7	
10	
15	
120	
0.1 N NaOH	

Calculation

Graph the volume of 0.1 N NaOH added (in drops) versus the pH of the mixture.

Cleanup Instruction

- Wash the glassware and return it to its proper location.

WRAP-UP

Conclusions

1. Do you think you could adjust the pH of a distilled water sample originally at pH of 7 to a pH of 8 using 0.1 N NaOH? Explain why.

2. Do you think you could adjust the pH of a distilled water sample originally at pH of 7 to a pH of 10 using 0.01 N NaOH? Explain why.

3. In which range would it be most difficult to adjust the pH of a distilled water sample to a specific pH value?

Challenge Questions and Extensions

4. Draw a graph similar to the one below using your data from this lab and Lab 6. Show the zero point at the center of the x-axis. The number of drops of HCl added begins at the zero point and increases to the left. The number of drops of NaOH added begins at the zero point and increases to the right.

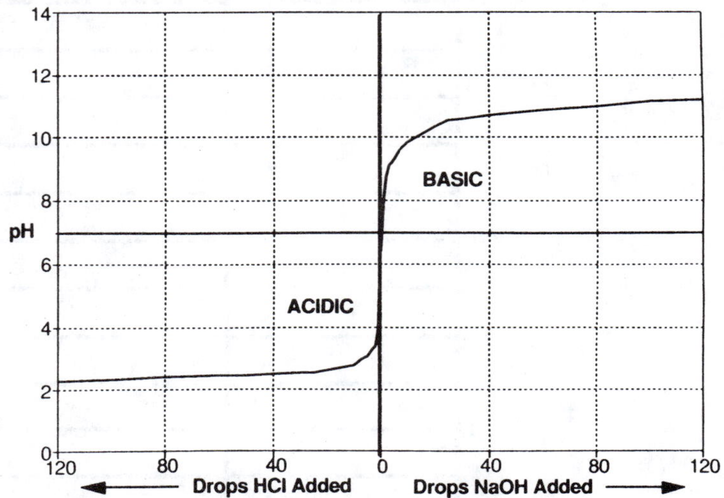

5. Start with a sample of 100 ml of freshly boiled distilled water. Add 120 drops of 0.1 N HCl to the water sample. Measure the pH of the mixture and then add drops of 0.1 N NaOH to the mixture. Begin by adding about 20 drops. When the pH change is more than 0.05 pH unit, decrease the number of drops by half—to 10, then to 5, then to 3, and finally to 1 drop between pH measurements. After the pH increases past a value of 7, the increases will decrease as before. When the pH change is less than 0.05 pH unit, double the number of drops added between measurements—1 drop, 3 drops, 5 drops, 10 drops, and 20 drops. When the pH change is less than 0.05 for an addition of 20 drops, or when a total of 240 drops of NaOH has been added, begin adding drops of HCl to the mixture. Begin with 20 drops as with the NaOH and use the same scheme used in adding the NaOH drops.

   Graph this data on two graphs—one showing the addition of NaOH, and the other showing the addition of HCl. (For the graph showing the addition of HCl, the drops of HCl added should increase to the left.) Compare the two graphs. How are they similar? How are they different?

Compare the two graphs to the graph of the data from Lab 6 and Lab 7. How are they similar? How are they different?

LAB 9

WHAT DO BUFFERS DO?

PREVIEW

Introduction

"Bob, the pH of Lake Pine Woods has been steadily dropping for the last 8 months," Gayle S. the acid rain technician told her supervisor. "The pH is approaching a point where we will begin to lose fish."

It sounds like it is time for a treatment with crushed limestone. We'll call and arrange for six flights tomorrow," Bob replied. "Watch the pH for two weeks after the treatment and let me know how it is doing."

Purpose

In this lab, you will titrate a weak acid solution (vinegar) with a strong base and observe the way the pH changes throughout the titration.

Lab Objectives

When you've finished this lab, you will be able to—

- Understand how buffers resist a pH change.
- Experimentally determine the pH range a buffer system can maintain.

Lab Skills

You will use these skills to complete this lab—

- Titrate a weak acid with a strong base.
- Measure the pH of a solution with pH paper or a pH meter.

Materials and Equipment Needed

250-ml beaker

0.1 N NaOH, 50 ml

vinegar, 25 ml

distilled water, freshly boiled, 25 ml

pH paper or pH meter

10-cc syringe

glass stirring rod

LAB PROCEDURE

Pre-Lab Discussion

A buffer is usually a weak acid and the salt of that weak acid and a strong base, or a weak base and the salt of that weak base and a strong acid.

The buffering of the lake with crushed limestone—primarily calcium carbonate ($CaCO_3$)—is a system between carbonic acid (H_2CO_3)—a weak acid—and calcium hydroxide ($Ca(OH)_2$)—a strong base. The reaction is—

$2H^+$	+	$CaCO_3$	→	H_2CO_3	+	Ca^{+2}
acid		calcium carbonate		carbonic acid		calcium ion

The acid is necessary for the calcium carbonate to dissolve. The carbonic acid is a weak acid and has a limited solubility in water. When the water becomes saturated with carbonic acid, the carbonic acid decomposes to water and carbon dioxide. If a base is added to this system, the hydroxide ions will react with the carbonic acid to from bicarbonate ion (HCO_3^-) and water. The secret of a buffer is that is has to have in solution, a substances that will react with acids or bases.

One way to study such a system is to begin with the weak acid and titrate (slowly add known volumes of a solution and monitor the change in the mixture) the solution with a strong base. In this lab, you will begin with vinegar—a solution of acetic acid. You will add a solution of sodium hydroxide to it in known increments and measure the pH after each addition.

Method

Put on your lab apron and goggles.

1. Pour 25 ml of the vinegar and 25 ml of freshly boiled distilled water into a 250-ml beaker.
2. Measure the pH of the vinegar solution with pH paper or a pH meter. Record the value in the Data Table.
3. Measure the pH of the 0.1 N NaOH. Record the value in the Data Table.

4. Add 10 cc of 0.1 N NaOH to the vinegar sample. Use the glass stirring rod to mix the sample. Measure the pH of the mixture and record the value in the Data Table.
5. Repeat step 4 until the pH of the vinegar sample begins to approach a pH of 10.

Data Table

0.1 N NaOH	
Volume of 0.1 NaOH Added (in cc)	**pH**
0	
10	
20	
30	
40	
50	
60	
70	
80	
90	
100	
110	
120	
130	
140	
150	
160	
170	
180	
190	
200	

Calculation

1. Graph pH versus volume of 0.1N NaOH added.

Cleanup Instructions

- Pour the solution from the beaker into the sink.
- Wash the glassware and return it to its proper place.

WRAP-UP

Conclusions

1. What pH range does the addition of NaOH have the smallest effect on the pH of the solution?
2. What do you think would be the pH range of an acetic acid/sodium acetate buffer system?

Challenge Questions and Extensions

3. Describe a method to experimentally determine the effective buffering pH range of an ammonium hydroxide/ammonium chloride (NH_4OH/NH_4Cl) buffer system?

SUBUNIT 5

How Can We Protect the Quality of Water?

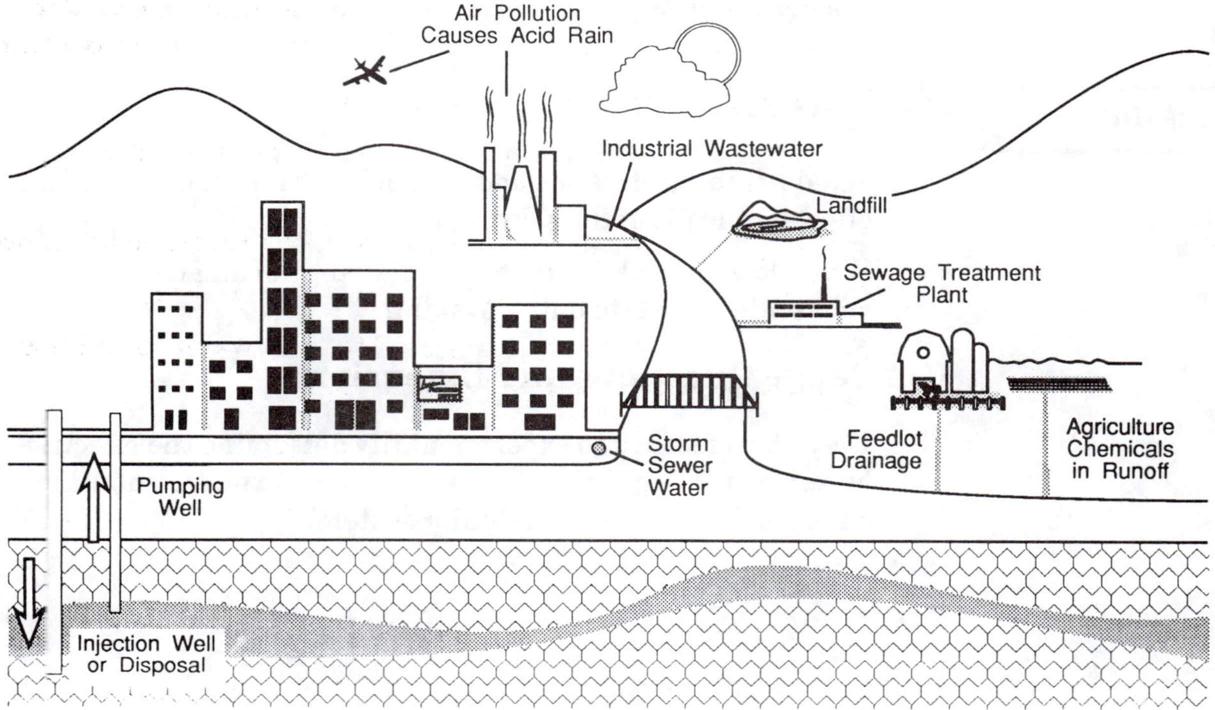

THINK ABOUT IT

- Which activities represented in the picture above have the greatest impact on water quality?
- How might you go about identifying the greatest sources of water pollution?
- What measures could be taken to minimize water pollution from the activities represented?
- How do you think the quality of the river water could be managed most effectively—through voluntary standards; federal laws, state laws or local laws; by media campaigns urging conservation and pollution prevention; or what other ways?

SUBUNIT OBJECTIVES

After you complete this subunit, you will be able to —

1. Analyze the relationship between water quality and water quantity.
2. Predict the potential impact on the quality of surface and/or groundwaters of at least seven different types of water pollution.
3. Identify the sources of water pollution.
4. Distinguish between point-source and nonpoint-source pollution.
5. Investigate five ways that pollution can be prevented or reduced.
6. Conduct at least four of seven tests of water quality.
7. Appraise the methods that are used to treat water to address different types of water-pollution problems.

How Does Pollution Enter the Water Cycle?

Win, Lose or Compromise?

Leroy and Veronica are sitting in the city council meeting room, waiting for the council meeting to begin. The room is packed with Save Hondo Springs activists. A small group of business development representatives is also present. Veronica recognizes a group from the local chapter of the Sierra Club.

"What's going to happen, do you think?" Veronica asks Lucy, the Sierra Club president.

"We think that the city staff is going to present a compromise ordinance," says Lucy. "It would limit the amount of impervious cover to 40%, would require all developments along the creek to collect the first quarter inch of rain runoff and treat it before allowing it to run into the creek. It won't allow for irrigation anywhere in the creek recharge zone, and

it reclassifies the golf course as a development. It also gets rid of exemptions for certain developers. Basically everybody would have to comply."

"That doesn't sound too bad," says Leroy. "Does the Sierra Club support it?"

"No," says Lucy. "We're pushing a counterproposal by Councilmember Lopez. He's calling for a 25% limit on impervious cover, treatment of 90% of all runoff—not just the first quarter inch of rainfall—and a few other minor differences." With that, Lucy is distracted by a fellow environmentalist and disappears into the crowd.

"Leroy, what is impervious cover?" asks Veronica quietly. "I can't remember."

"Parking lots, rooftops, roads, anything that keeps water from soaking through," responds Leroy.

"40% seems high, then," Veronica says. "Still, all this is sounding a little better than before, when it looked like there weren't going to be any restrictions at all."

"Yeah," says Leroy, "sometimes you win, sometimes you lose, sometimes you compromise."

"Well, in this case, a compromise is the same as losing," says a voice behind them. They turn to see one of the Save Hondo Springs activists. Veronica and Leroy look at one another with raised eyebrows.

"Is that true?" asks Leroy.

But by now the council has assembled, the mayor has opened the meeting, and the third round of hearings is under way.

At the beginning of this unit, you read about the water cycle. The water cycle restores water supplies that are lost in evaporation, runoff and human use. However, as water moves continuously among rivers and oceans, land and the atmosphere, it can become contaminated, or polluted, by unwanted materials. To understand how this occurs, let's review the water cycle (Figure 5-1) and consider how pollution could occur throughout the cycle.

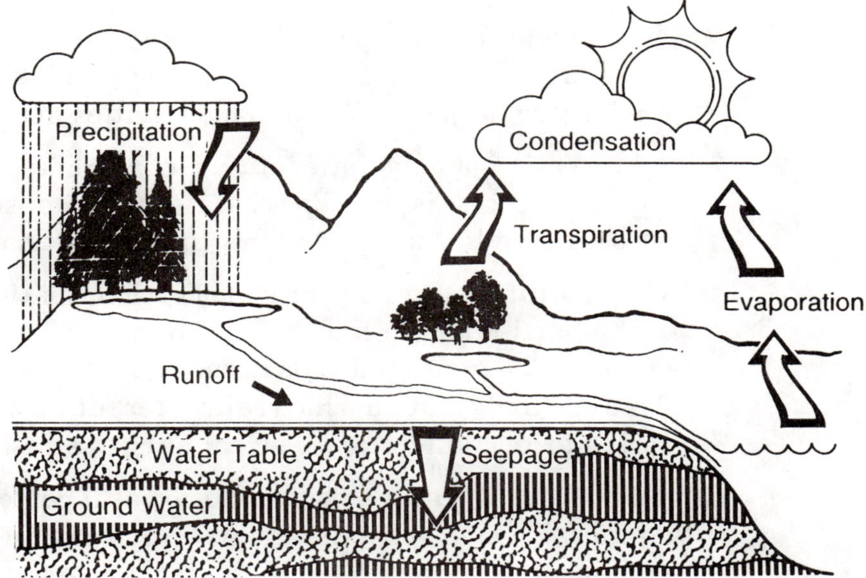

Figure 5-1
The water cycle

Evaporation

Water from oceans, rivers, other surface waters, and the leaves of plants evaporates and becomes part of the atmosphere. Water vapor in the atmosphere interacts with other chemicals in the air, such as sulfur oxides and nitrogen oxides that are emitted by automobiles or industries.

Condensation and Precipitation

Water vapor eventually **condenses**; that is, it changes to a liquid again as it is cooled in the atmosphere. It falls to Earth as **precipitation** (rain or ice). If it has formed compounds with harmful chemicals in the atmosphere, the compounds will fall as contaminated precipitation, such as acid rain. As water vapor condenses into rain or ice, it can also bring with it airborne particulates—dusts of metals and other materials.

Runoff and Percolation

When water falls to Earth as rain or ice, it flows over the surface of the land, eventually reaching **surface waters:** streams, lakes and rivers. The water that flows over the land is called **runoff**. Runoff is vulnerable to pollution because it can pick up soil, harmful chemicals, and organic wastes as it moves across the land. Runoff carries its contaminants into the body of surface water into which it flows.

A **watershed** is the total drainage area from which runoff water flows to a common point such as a river or a lake. Water pollution often occurs as a result of human activities in the watershed.

Water not only flows into rivers and lakes, it also goes into the soil; this process is called **percolation**. Water seeps downward through Earth's surface and into groundwater aquifers.

Aquifers are sand, gravel or rock formations below the surface of the Earth that are saturated with water. The water found within cracks and porous materials in the aquifer is called **groundwater**. Areas of land through which rainwater filters down through soil and rock into an aquifer are called **recharge zones**.

Water is vulnerable to pollution as it percolates downward to the aquifer. Human activities that take place in the recharge zone have an impact on the quality of the water that goes into the aquifer. Water can carry contaminants with it down to the aquifer. Materials other than water, such as chemicals from leaking storage tanks or landfills, can percolate into the aquifer, too.

Withdrawal and Use of Water for Human Activities

In most parts of Earth, human beings have become an important part of the water cycle. We withdraw surface water and groundwater to use for energy production, manufacturing, irrigating crops, drinking and sanitation. Water withdrawals nearly always reenter the water cycle at a later time, but usually the quality of the water has been altered, or polluted, in some way. Often substances have been added to it: salt, nutrients, metals, organic materials, and other toxins. Sometimes the temperature has been raised. In some cases, water has become radioactive. For the rest of this subunit, we will look at how water is polluted by various human activities, how pollution can be prevented, and how used water, or wastewater, can be treated to improve its quality.

Water Quality and Water Quantity

As the world population grows and water withdrawals increase, the question comes up: Is there enough water on Earth to meet our needs? The answer is not simple. Because water cycles throughout the environment, it is a renewable resource. However, water withdrawals that are polluted during use and left untreated or inadequately treated will carry contaminants throughout the cycle. As a result, water may be available, but it may also be unsuitable for many purposes: drinking, bathing, recreation, certain types of industrial processing, and energy production, to name a few. Pollution of surface water and groundwater eventually makes fresh, usable water more difficult to acquire. So water quality affects water availability, or water quantity.

Water quantity can also have an effect on water quality. When groundwater is withdrawn over a period of time at a faster rate than it can be replenished, a condition called **overdraft** occurs. In areas in which saltwater sources are nearby, overdraft can lead to the intrusion of salt water into freshwater aquifers.

JOB PROFILE: HYDROGRAPHIC SURVEY TECHNICIAN

Steven R. is a hydrographic survey technician who works for a university research station. He surveys and gathers data in the tidal and coastal areas of his state on the East Coast.

"I work as part of a research team. We gather data for a lot of different projects, but almost all of them have to do with the water quality and movement in the wetlands and coastal region of the state. These tidal flats and marshes are very important to our water supply and water quality. They are spawning areas for fish and habitats for many species of wildlife."

Steve operates standard surveying instruments such as sextants (instruments for measuring distances), depth recorders, wire drags and navigational instruments. He has to read charts and help the team's cartographer (mapmaker) in the field.

Steve explains that the team monitors the wetlands and the coastal region. "We look at where the water is moving, especially as development increases in this area. We also monitor groundwater quality. In coastal regions like this one, we are concerned about overdraft. If overdraft should occur, our groundwater supply would be subject to saltwater intrusion."

Steve likes his job. "I really like to be out here working," he says simply. "The marshes and the tidal flats are full of life."

What Are the Kinds of Water Pollution?

How do we define what is a pollutant and what is not? The Clean Water Act (a law passed by the U.S. Congress in 1974 and renewed in 1987) defines "pollution" as the "man-made or man-induced alteration of the chemical, physical, biological and radiological integrity of the water." Major pollutants are listed and discussed below.

Salt

Most water, even fresh water, contains some salt. Some industries produce wastewater with a high salt content. The use of water for crop irrigation in areas where drainage is poor can lead to increased salt concentrations. Some irrigation water evaporates and some is taken up by plants. The remaining water is left with a higher concentration of salt, which can eventually leach down to groundwater.

Whatever its cause, excess salt in groundwater—if the groundwater is pumped for further irrigation—can eventually stunt plants or kill them. Excessive salt can also make water unfit for drinking.

Toxic Substances

Toxic substances are substances that are harmful to human and animal health. The term toxic is usually reserved for those substances that are harmful in low concentrations, for example, heavy metals such as mercury, cadmium and lead and organic chemicals such as benzene, chloroform, nitrosamines, and polychlorinated biphenyls (PCBs). Some toxic substances may cause immediate damage to body tissues and functions. Others may be factors in causing cancer, or may cause other diseases if exposure continues over a long period of time.

Organic Wastes

Organic wastes come from human and animal sewage, wood and paper mills, food processing and numerous other sources. When organic wastes decay in water, water is robbed of dissolved oxygen. Organic wastes also pollute water by adding solid materials to it.

Sediment

Sediment is any solid material that settles out of a solution. Sediment pollution often occurs in nature. For example, heavy rains and flooding can cause the eventual filling in of riverbeds with fine sediment known as silt. Sediment is also often produced by agricultural operations, construction activities, and logging and forestry operations. Sediment causes water to become cloudy and can impede the flow of water. It can also block fish gills and hinder respiration in other aquatic species.

Acids

Acids are produced as a by-product of mining and many industrial operations. Most aquatic life must have an environmental pH of at least 5 to 6 in order to survive, so acid wastes can be very harmful. Humans have to keep the pH of their internal body fluids very near the neutral point and cannot drink highly acidic water.

Bacteria and Viruses

Bacteria and viruses are found in human and animal wastes. Left untreated, such wastes can cause diseases. One indicator of the presence of bacteria and viruses is the total coliform count. If coliform bacteria are present in high numbers, it is assumed that disease-causing bacteria are present.

Nutrients

Nutrients such as phosphorus and nitrogen might be expected to be a good thing, but excessive amounts in water can cause too much plant and algae growth. When these plants and algae decay, the bacteria that decompose them consume oxygen needed by fish and other aquatic life.

Oil and Grease

Oil spills in ocean waters are fatal to many marine animals and plants, both in the water and along the coastline. Oil interferes with gas exchange at the surface of the water. It can coat marine animals, interfering with respiration, temperature regulation, and mobility. Also, some compounds in oil are toxic.

Heat

Water is used as a coolant in power plants and some industrial processes. If high-temperature cooling water is released into surface waters, it reduces oxygen solubility, thereby making it impossible for many species of fish and wildlife to live in the water. By contrast, the direct effect of the heat is not usually a major problem, especially if the discharge water comes to equilibrium with a large body of water.

Activity 5-1

This activity is best carried out by a group of two to four students.

- Contact your local electrical power plant and arrange to interview the supervisor of plant operations or an environmental technician who works for the plant.
- Find out what happens to water that has been used as a coolant for power plant processes. Is it cooled before being released to local surface waters? If so, how?
- Find out about other water treatment processes in the power plant. Which uses of water require water of the greatest purity? Why?
- Find out how many people who work in the power plant are involved primarily with water treatment.
- Share your information with the class.

Radioactivity

A variety of activities in the medical field (certain diagnostic materials and radiation therapy), energy production (nuclear power production) and the defense industry (nuclear weapons) generate radioactive wastes, including water that has become radioactive. Safe storage of such wastes presents many problems.

Radioactive materials may be harmful to organisms when they give off ionizing radiation. Ionizing radiation can damage the complex molecules that make up cells and tissues.

What Processes Cause Water To Become Polluted?

Water can be contaminated in three main ways:

- Through natural processes
- Through human waste-disposal practices
- Through accidental leaks and spills or other unplanned, unforeseen contamination

Natural Processes of Water Pollution

Some natural processes change the composition of water. **Leaching** is the process by which water carries dissolved or suspended materials as it percolates down to the groundwater. Leaching can carry minerals that, although they occur naturally in the soil, are not desirable to have in groundwater in excessive amounts. Some naturally occurring chemicals that can cause problems in water quality include chlorides, sulfates, nitrates and arsenic. Leaching can also carry radioactivity from uranium deposits.

Other natural processes that cause water pollution are storms and flooding. Floodwaters can erode soil, carrying it into surface waters.

Waste-Disposal Practices as a Cause of Pollution

The waste-disposal practices of humans are a major source of water pollution. Waste disposal occurs in the following situations:

- Municipal and privately owned sewage systems
- Landfills for the disposal of solid wastes
- Industrial wastewater discharges
- Sludge disposal (Sludge is the solid residue of wastewater treatment.)
- Brine disposal (strong salt solutions, associated especially with the petroleum industry)
- Disposal of mine wastes
- Animal feedlot wastes
- High- and low-level radioactive wastes from medical, energy and defense activities

Pollution can occur with any of the waste-disposal activities listed above if waste is untreated or improperly treated, or if it is improperly stored or discharged.

Some of these wastes include natural and synthetic chemicals that have a major impact on water quality. One study estimated that as of 1980, over thirty thousand chemicals were being used and distributed throughout the environment, and that a thousand new chemicals were being added each year. Whether these go down the drain, into a river or ocean, into the air, or into a landfill, they are part of the waste generated by human activities.

Activity 5-2

This activity is best carried out by a group of two to four students.

- Contact your town's solid waste department manager. Arrange for an interview.
- Find out how solid waste is disposed of in your community. Are there provisions for recycling? What kinds of wastes are allowed or disallowed in the local landfills? Are there special provisions for disposal of hazardous chemicals by domestic and business users?
- Find out what features of the landfill help to protect against groundwater contamination.
- Report your findings to the class.

Leaks, Spills and Other Unplanned Water Contamination

A third source of water pollution includes accidental spills of hazardous wastes, leaks from storage tanks and wells, and other unplanned or unforeseen contamination. Crop farming, mining, and highway deicing are examples of activities that can cause significant pollution of surface water and groundwater. In these cases, pollution does not occur as a result of waste disposal, but as a result of the process itself. Automobile emissions might fall into this category. We don't normally think that we are disposing of "petrochemical wastes" as we drive our cars, but we are leaving an exhaust trail in the air that contributes to acid rain.

JOB PROFILE: HYDROGEOLOGIST

Christa P. is a hydrogeologist who works for a civil engineering firm. The firm does environmental studies for businesses and government agencies.

"A hydrogeologist has to incorporate a basic understanding of groundwater flow with a knowledge of geology and chemistry," says Christa. "Much of my work involves helping companies comply with environmental regulations. For example, we might be called out to evaluate groundwater if a company's underground storage tanks were suspected of leakage. Or we might be hired to routinely monitor the groundwater in the tank storage area."

When asked what steps she would take in such a situation, Christa explains, "We install monitoring wells—these are small-diameter pipes that are placed into the ground. Groundwater comes up into the pipe, and we're able to sample it. We also do soil borings and test soil for contamination. If we find contamination, we help the company make a plan to remedy the situation. But prevention is always better than remediation."

What Are the Sources of Water Pollution?

People who track down water pollution separate its sources into two groups: point-source pollution and nonpoint-source pollution. Point-source pollution includes material that is discharged directly from a specific source. Nonpoint-source includes runoff from sources that are more widespread and harder to identify: city streets, fields of crops. Table 5-1 lists sources of point-source and nonpoint-source pollution. Note that some of the sources are sites of waste treatment or storage. They can become sources of pollution if waste treatment or storage is inadequate.

Table 5-1. Sources of Water Pollution—Point and Nonpoint

Point-source pollution	Nonpoint-source pollution
Municipal sewage-treatment plant discharges (where treatment is inadequate)	Stormwater runoff
Industrial discharges (where treatment is inadequate)	Atmospheric contaminants
Leaking underground storage tanks	Leaching waste disposal sites
Feedlots and manure storage (if improperly maintained)	Leaching agricultural chemicals
Some stormwater discharges	Sludge (if improperly treated) disposal
	Failing septic tanks
	Leaking landfills or dumps
	Marine sources (ocean dumping and other waste disposal)
	Land-use decisions (loss of wetland or vegetative cover, increased paved surfaces)
	Abandoned mine drainage

In Subunit 3, you read about three groups of water users: domestic, agricultural, and industrial. Let's look again at these three groups to see how each one contributes to water pollution problems. The graph in Figure 5-2 shows the percentage of wastewater produced by each group. The graph shows a fourth group, steam electric power generation, which heads the list of wastewater producers. However, keep in mind that most water used in the steam electric power industry is for cooling purposes and is returned to its source with few or no added pollutants. Boiler-cleaning operations in steam power plants do produce some toxic pollutants.

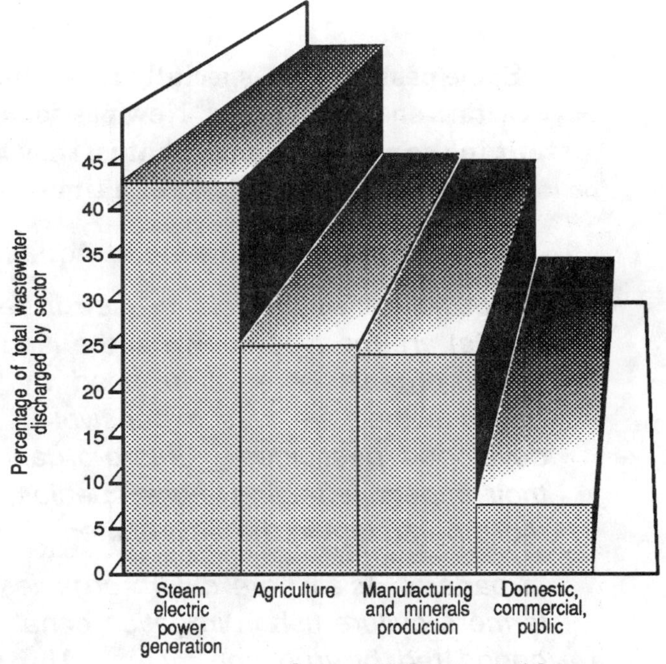

Figure 5-2
U.S. wastewater discharges

Water Pollution from Agricultural Sources

There are three main agricultural sources of water pollution: agrochemicals, irrigation, and feedlot operations.

Agrochemicals

Most crop farmers routinely use **agrochemicals** to promote the growth and health of field crops. These chemicals include fertilizers and pesticides. Pesticides include herbicides (chemicals that control or destroy weed growth), insecticides (chemicals that control or destroy insect populations) and fungicides (chemicals that control or destroy unwanted fungi).

Fertilizers. Fertilizer runoff can cause increases in the nitrate and phosphate pollution of some water supplies. It can also speed up a natural process called eutrophication that occurs in surface waters. **Eutrophication** is a part of the normal aging process of lakes. As a lake ages, its content of organic matter increases. The organic matter settles and fills in the bottom (of the lake). As the organic matter decays, a large share of the lake's oxygen is consumed. Surface waters polluted by excess nutrients and organic matter eventually become oxygen-starved, and species that require oxygen die out.

Pesticides. The seriousness of water pollution caused by pesticides depends on several factors: how quickly a particular pesticide breaks down in the environment, how many species of organisms it affects, and how it is used.

Some pesticides—especially recently developed ones—target only certain species of pests. New pesticides also tend to be less **persistent** in the environment. That is, they break down into harmless or less harmful components after a time.

Pesticide Use Threatens Aquaculture Operations

About half of all pesticides used in less-developed countries (LDCs) are the type known in the industry as chloro-organics. Chloro-organics are often used by the farmers of LDCs because they are less expensive than some of the recently developed pesticides. Chloro-organics also are broader in their impact (affecting more species), more destructive, and more persistent in the environment.

In parts of Asia where chloro-organics are in wide use, many farmers culture fish in irrigation canals, in rice paddies and in ponds fed by irrigation water. The use of chloro-organics, which persist and accumulate in water systems long after use, is threatening these aquaculture operations. Having recognized that moderately high concentrations of chloro-organics kill fish, many farmers are reluctant to invest in fry (newly hatched fishes) for their paddies or ponds. They fear that lingering pesticide pollution will kill the stock.

As you can see from the scenario above, a broadly powerful, persistent pesticide can pollute water supplies to the point of causing fish kills. Pesticides can kill off algae and other plant life, which in turn, degrades the quality of surface waters. The uptake of pesticides, by producers in an aquatic food chain contributes to the buildup of pesticides in animals along the food chain.

Some pesticides, if present in high enough concentrations, can be harmful to human health. They may cause sterility or birth defects; they may be a factor in causing cancer; they may cause other health problems. In the past, the Environmental Protection Agency has banned the use of certain pesticides on some crops because they have been proven harmful in field studies and/or laboratory tests.

The potential of fertilizers and pesticides to pollute water depends on many variables. Just mentioned was the factor of **persistence** (taking a long time to break down). Another factor is the water solubility of a compound. The greater the **water solubility** of the pesticide or fertilizer, the more likely it is to reach groundwater. Some chemicals have a property of strong **soil adsorption** (attachment to soil particles) and are less likely to move into groundwater. In addition, the soil texture and composition and the underlying geology of the region have an effect on how agrochemicals will behave.

One of the most important factors in water pollution caused by agrochemicals is how the chemicals are applied. When such chemicals are applied in proper amounts, with attention to timing, weather conditions, and other environmental factors, their pollution effects can be minimized. If they are used carelessly or overused, they can cause significant contamination. In considering how agrochemicals are applied, we have to be aware that the use of agrochemicals is not limited to farmers. Landscapers, groundskeepers, golf-course maintenance workers, and many, many individuals use pesticides and fertilizers on their lawns, grounds and gardens.

Activity 5-3

- Contact a person from one of the occupations listed: farmers, landscapers, groundskeepers, golf-course maintenance workers, home gardeners, plant nursery managers.
- Ask each person the same set of questions:
  1. Do you use fertilizers and pesticides in your growing or maintenance operations?
  2. If yes, what kinds and for what purposes?
  3. How are the fertilizers and pesticides applied?
  4. Do you take precautions in your application of fertilizers and pesticides?
  5. If yes, what kind of precautions?
  6. Do you take any precautions that are designed to protect the water supply?
- Share your information with the class. There should be at least four interviews in each occupational category if everyone in the class participates. Discuss whether different groups appear to have different attitudes and/or practices in their use of agrochemicals. If so, what are they?

Irrigation

Irrigation accounts for the greatest share of water use in agriculture. Irrigation can contribute to an increase in water salinity, especially in areas where drainage is poor. As explained earlier, when irrigation water evaporates or is taken up by plants, the soil is left with a higher concentration of salt, which can eventually leach down to groundwater or become part of surface-water runoff. The inability of most plants and animals to tolerate water that has an excessive salt content was discussed earlier in this subunit.

Irrigation can also be a problem when it leads to overdraft of groundwater. (Remember from earlier in this subunit that overdraft is the withdrawal of groundwater at a rate faster than it can be replenished.) Overdraft, in turn, can lead to a collapse of surface land called **subsidence** as well as **saltwater intrusion**, also discussed earlier.

Feedlot Operations

Forty years ago, feedlots were rare. Livestock and even poultry ranged over large land areas, and their wastes naturally recycled to the soil. For example, the ratio of land to steer was around 8600 square feet per steer in many cattle-raising operations. Today the ratio is 35 to 200 square feet per steer. Therefore, manure from animal populations has become a significant factor in wastewater management. The problem is even greater because of the increased use of commercial chemical fertilizers among farmers. Farmers who in the past might have used manure to fertilize fields no longer recycle feedlot wastes.

Over the last twenty years, legislation has been passed to limit feedlot operations. As a result, groundwater contamination from feedlot operations is not as great a threat as it used to be. More problematic is the pollution of surface waters by feedlot wastes. Especially with heavy rains, runoff can pollute surface waters, causing the following problems:

- Increased oxygen-demanding wastes
- Increased eutrophication of surface waters, from increased nitrates and especially, increased phosphates
- Fish kills
- Bacterial contamination harmful to humans

Water Pollution from Industrial Sources

As you read in Subunit 3, industries use water to produce energy, to transport raw materials, to cool industrial equipment, to lubricate materials and equipment, to clean and finish, and as an ingredient in a product. The wastewater produced by some industries is contaminated with toxic substances that require specialized treatment and waste storage. If treatment is inadequate, these industries can be major polluters. Industries may contribute to pollution through inadequate storage and handling of materials that make up their products or that are used in processing. For example, a company that uses a large amount of acid in its operation may store the acid in underground storage tanks. If the tanks are not properly constructed, installed or maintained and begin to leak, then groundwater pollution can result.

Table 5-2 lists some industries that produce contaminated wastewater that requires one or more types of treatment before it can be released. The wastewater discharges of these (and other) industries are regulated by law and monitored by the U.S. Environmental Protection Agency. Table 5-3 lists industrial wastewater pollutants that are monitored by the Environmental Protection Agency, as of this writing.

Table 5-2: Industries Whose Wastewater Discharge Is Regulated

Adhesives	Porcelain enamel	Pharmaceuticals
Leather tanning and finishing	Gum and wood chemicals	Plastic and synthetic materials
Soaps and detergents	Paint and ink	Rubber
Aluminum-forming	Printing and publishing	Auto and other laundries
Battery manufacturing	Pulp and paper	Mechanical products
Coil coating	Textile mills	Electric and electronic components
Copper-forming	Timber	Explosives manufacturing
Electroplating	Coal mining	Inorganic chemicals
Foundries	Ore mining	
Iron and steel	Petroleum refining	
Nonferrous metals	Steam electric	
Photographic supplies	Organic chemicals	
Plastics processing	Pesticides	

Source: U.S. Environmental Protection Agency

Table 5-3: Priority Industrial Wastewater Pollutants

Acenapthene	DDT and metabolites	Nitrobenzene
Acrolein	Dichlorobenzenes	Nitrophenols
Acrylonitrile	Dichlorobenzidine	Nitrosamines
Aldrin/dieldrin	Dichloroethylenes	Pentachlorophenol
Antimony and compounds	2, 4-Dimethylphenol	Phenol
Arsenic and compounds	Dinitrotoluene	Phthalate esters
Asbestos	Diphenylhydrazine	Polychlorinated biphenyls (PCBs)
Benzene	Endosulfan and metabolites	Polynuclear aromatic hydrocarbons
Benzidine	Endrin and metabolites	Selenium and compounds
Beryllium and compounds	Ethylbenzene	Silver and compounds
Cadmium and compounds	Fluoranthene	2, 3, 7, 8 - Tetrachlorodibenzo- *p*-dioxin (TCDD)
Carbon tetrachloride	Haloethers	Tetrachloroethylene
Chlordane	Halomethanes	Thallium and compounds
Chlorinated benzenes	Heptachlor and metabolites	Toluene
Chlorinated ethanes	Hexachlorobutadiene	Toxaphene
Chloralkyl ethers	Hexachlorocyclopentadiene	Trichloroethylene
Chlorinated phenols	Hexachlorocyclohexane	Vinyl chloride
Chloroform	Isophorone	Zinc and compounds
2-Chlorophenol	Lead and compounds	
Chromium and compounds	Mercury and compounds	
Copper and compounds	Naphthalene	
Cyanides	Nickel and compounds	

Source: U.S. Environmental Protection Agency

Figure 5-3 distinguishes between total waste production and hazardous waste production in industry. The graph is based on a 1981 Environmental Protection Agency study, which identified 60,000 firms that have the potential to generate hazardous waste. The gray areas of the graph show the portion of waste that is poisonous, corrosive, disease-causing, burnable or otherwise hazardous.

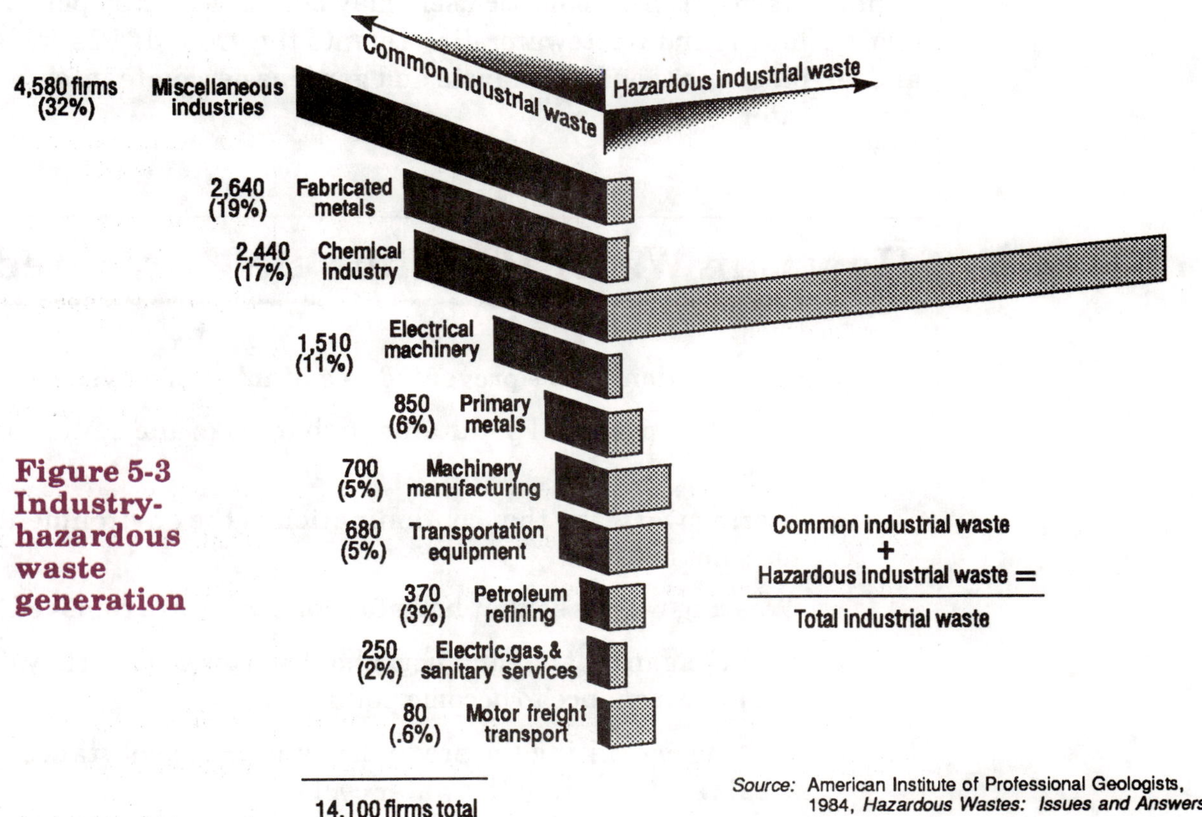

Figure 5-3 Industry-hazardous waste generation

Source: American Institute of Professional Geologists, 1984, *Hazardous Wastes: Issues and Answers.*

Activity 5-4

In small groups of three or four students, analyze the graph in Figure 5-3 to answer the following questions: Which type of industry appears to generate the greatest amount of hazardous material? Which type of industry appears to generate the greatest amount of general wastes?

Water Pollution from Domestic Sources

All of us are domestic users of water; we use water for drinking, cleaning, and flushing body wastes. Most people's personal wastewater goes into a municipal water system. If we pour toxic chemicals down the sink, they go into that system, too. Commercial businesses that use municipal water systems are included in the category of domestic users, as are public buildings. In rural areas, many people have single-family septic systems to handle wastes.

In addition to domestic wastewater that goes into a municipal system or septic tank, domestic users may pollute water by pouring oils, chemicals and wastewater directly into the ground. Pesticides and fertilizers used on home lawns and gardens percolate into groundwater.

How Can Water Pollution Be Prevented?

Water pollution can be prevented in a number of ways:

- Handling potential pollutants so that leaks and spills do not occur
- Storing wastes so that contamination of the environment does not result
- Treating wastes so that harmful pollutants are removed
- Recycling industrial and household wastes so that they do not have a chance to become pollutants
- Halting or limiting the production and use of substances that are likely to get into the water cycle
- Minimizing the amount of water used in a process or activity

Let's look at some examples of success in three areas: in agriculture, industry and the community at large.

Water-Pollution Prevention in Agriculture

One way crop growers prevent or reduce the pollution of groundwater is to use fertilizers and pesticides sparingly, providing crops with the lowest dose that is effective. New pesticides have been developed that are effective in very low concentrations. For example, in the 1950s use rates for herbicides were typically ten pounds per acre of cropland. Today, a ten-pound application of one of the newly developed herbicides (one group is called sulfonylureas) can control weeds on several thousand acres of cropland.

Proper handling of agricultural chemicals can also greatly reduce pollution of groundwater. In using crop chemicals, farmers, and other crop growers should observe the following guidelines:

- Make sure spraying equipment is operating properly and is free of leaks.
- Avoid contamination from backsiphoning (chemicals allowed to back up into the water supply).
- After spraying, rinse chemical containers and add the rinse water to the spray tank for reuse.
- Store chemicals away from surface waters and wells and ensure their containers are not leaking.

Activity 5-5

You are part of the package-design team working for the manufacturer of a potentially harmful insecticide spray. Design a product label that will help users of the insecticide to keep from contaminating water supplies.

Since agricultural activities account for nearly one-half of freshwater use in the U.S., minimizing water use is very important in maintaining water quality. A number of methods, some based on advanced technologies, are now being used to increase the efficiency of irrigation.

A system of irrigation called drip, or trickle, irrigation can greatly improve the efficiency of water use, especially in dry climates. In drip irrigation, water is applied directly to each crop plant through a network of plastic pipes with holes at intervals along the pipe surface. Drip irrigation cuts water use greatly from conventional sprinkler irrigation.

Drip irrigation is most efficient when farmland is completely level. In some areas of the U.S., farmland is leveled to within one inch of smoothness using **laser technology**. A laser-sending unit at the edge of a field sends a signal to a tractor, and the depth of the tractor's scrapers is adjusted accordingly to move earth from high spots to fill in low spots.

Some sprinkler irrigation systems are controlled by computers. Sensing units in fields relay data to the computer on factors such as soil moisture. The computer responds by releasing the required amount of water to the sprinkling system in areas where water is needed.

Another efficient method of watering some types of crops involves increasing the depth of tillable soil. This practice boosts the availability of soil water to plants by slowing the downward percolation of water. As a result, more plants can be set per row. This not only improves per acre yields, but the closer spacing of crop plants means that weeds are not able to compete well with crops for soil water.

Water-Pollution Prevention in Industry

Many industries are required by law to pretreat wastewater from manufacturing plants before it enters municipal sewage systems. Pretreatment reduces the amount of pollutants that enters the waste stream and decreases the overall burden on municipal systems.

Through the Toxic Substances Control Act, the U.S. Environmental Protection Agency has the power to prohibit or limit production, use, storage, distribution and disposal of substances that present a significant health risk. Toxic substances called PCBs (polychlorinated biphenyls) are just one example of a chemical hazard whose use has been eliminated. These substances, once commonly used in electrical transformers, had been getting into rivers and harbors and seriously affecting water quality. Unfortunately, many other substances that pose substantial health risks remain in use. These are often disposed of at sites where leaching into groundwater can occur.

An industrial management strategy called **in-process recycling** is helping to reduce wastes in a number of industries. As a result of in-process recycling, wastes from one point in a production process are cycled back into the process for reuse. In the printing industry, for example, inks dissolved in toxic organic solvents—if spilled—can pollute the environment. Through in-process recycling, nearly all of the solvent is recycled rather than discarded as hazardous waste.

Other waste-reduction techniques now being initiated in some industries include:

- Replacing raw materials with alternatives that do not produce pollutants
- Improving plant operations to reduce leaks and spills of potential pollutants
- Modifying the product or the production process so that polluting substances are not used

Water-Pollution Prevention in the Community and the Home

End Grime with Enzymes

Calvin L. is a marketing representative for a large detergent manufacturer. His company has just developed a new soap formula for cleaning clothes. The new product will not only clean better but will produce less waste.

Calvin explains, "Our slogan for selling our new line of laundry detergents is 'End grime with enzymes.' The key to our new soap formula is the replacement of stain-removing compounds in the soap with natural substances called enzymes. Enzymes are substances made by living organisms and used to speed up their biochemical reactions. One way that enzymes do this is by binding large molecules and breaking them into smaller molecules. This is also how enzymes function in the washing machine. Enzymes bind to substances responsible for tough stains, such as those produced by soil, and break them apart.

"One advantage to using enzymes in detergents is that enzymes are highly effective in small quantities. Detergent enzymes aren't destroyed or absorbed during washing. They work over and over. Much less enzyme is needed in a soap formula than traditional stain remover. So wash water entering the sewage lines is much less concentrated in water pollutants than if a conventional detergent were used.

"Another advantage is that many commercial enzymes can now be produced through biotechnology. This means that the cells of microorganisms living in laboratory vats are producing enzymes through their natural processes. This is not only less costly than trying to make synthetic enzymes in

a laboratory but requires fewer raw materials, again less waste produced overall.

"Right now our R & D team is trying to discover an enzyme that could bleach your clothes during the wash cycle. This would mean we could do away with bleaching agents in our products, reducing water pollution even further."

Pollution studies are showing that for some types of water pollutants, domestic polluters contribute as much as industrial and agricultural polluters do. Many neighborhoods and communities around the nation are taking important steps to reduce or prevent pollution. A number of cities have placed restrictions on the types of materials that can be accepted at landfills. A number of recycling centers encourage the drop-off of hazardous chemicals that are used around the home. Such chemicals include cleaning compounds, automotive fluids, lawn and garden chemicals, etc.

Activity 5-6

- Obtain a recent water bill for your residence. Determine from the bill the number of gallons of water your household used for the billing period and the total charge for water used.
- Call the water company to find out how the total charge was calculated.
- List ways that your household could reduce its water bill. Consider water used in the kitchen, bathroom, and laundry room, as well as outside the house itself.

How Is Water Quality Tested?

Water-quality testing at a water or wastewater treatment plant is required by law. Numerous types of tests are done on samples of water taken before, during, and after treatment. (Some of the more common treatment methods for wastewater are discussed later in this section.) Such tests monitor not only water quality but the effectiveness of the treatment process. Right now, let's survey six tests routinely carried out at treatment plants. Some of the tests may also be used in other situations, such as pool and spa care.

Testing for Total Solids

Most of the pollutants in a water supply are actually solids. The smallest solids are either in suspension or are dissolved. Together these are referred to as total solids. Both suspended and dissolved solids may be either organic or inorganic. Organic solids constitute the bulk of wastewater pollution.

To determine the total solids in a sample of wastewater, a wastewater-treatment technician transfers a well-mixed water sample to an evaporating dish whose weight is known very precisely. The dish with sample is dried in an oven at 103°C for one hour. After drying, the dish is weighed on a precision balance. The amount of total solids in the water sample are determined as:

$$\text{Total solids} = \text{Weight of dish with sample after drying} - \text{Weight of dish}$$

Equation 5-1

Testing for Organic and Inorganic Solids

The test for organic and inorganic solids in a water sample is carried out immediately following the test for total solids. In this test, the dish containing total solids of the sample is placed in a special furnace at 600°C for 15 minutes. (It is assumed that all organics will **volatilize** at this temperature. Inorganics will remain behind in the dish.) After cooling and redrying at 103°C the dish with sample is weighed. The amount of organic solids is determined as follows:

$$\text{Organic solids} = \text{Weight of dish holding total solids} - \text{Weight of dish with solids after vaporizing and redrying}$$

Equation 5-2

The amount of inorganic solids can be calculated at the same time the amount of organic solids is calculated. The formula for inorganic solids is:

$$\text{Inorganic solids} = \text{Total solids} - \text{Organic solids}$$

Equation 5-3

Activity 5-7

A wastewater-treatment technician places an evaporating dish (weight = 40.0000 g) containing a 100-ml water sample into a drying oven set at 103°C. After one hour the technician removes the dish and records the weight of dish plus sample as 40.1010 g.

- Find the total solids in the sample in mg/liter.

The technician now places the dried sample into a 600°C furnace to vaporize all organic matter. After fifteen minutes she removes the dish and cools and redries it at 103°C. The dish with remaining sample is then put on a balance and found to weigh 40.0505 g.

- Find the organic solids and inorganic solids in the sample in mg/liter.

Dissolved Oxygen Tests

A number of factors influence the amount of oxygen gas in a sample of water, including temperature and the amount of other dissolved materials in the water. Microbes in water use dissolved oxygen, or dO_2, during respiration (by oxidation). In fact, dissolved oxygen can become depleted when there is a heavy load of oxidizable material in the water. This takes place because the microbes are oxidizing the large amounts of organic solids present.

Dissolved-oxygen levels can be measured in two ways: 1) with a special probe attached to a meter, and 2) through a series of chemical reactions called the **Winkler Method**.

A dissolved-oxygen probe, shown in Figure 5-4, contains a pair of **electrodes** in a current-carrying solution. When the probe is placed in a sample of water, the electrodes are kept from direct contact with the sample by a synthetic membrane (often made of Teflon). Oxygen, however, can pass through this membrane from the water sample into the electrode solution. As the oxygen enters the solution it is reduced (gains electrons). This reduction causes a very small current to flow in the electrode solution. The current may be read from a meter attached to the probe. The amount of dO_2 originally in the water is directly related to the amount of current flow in the solution.

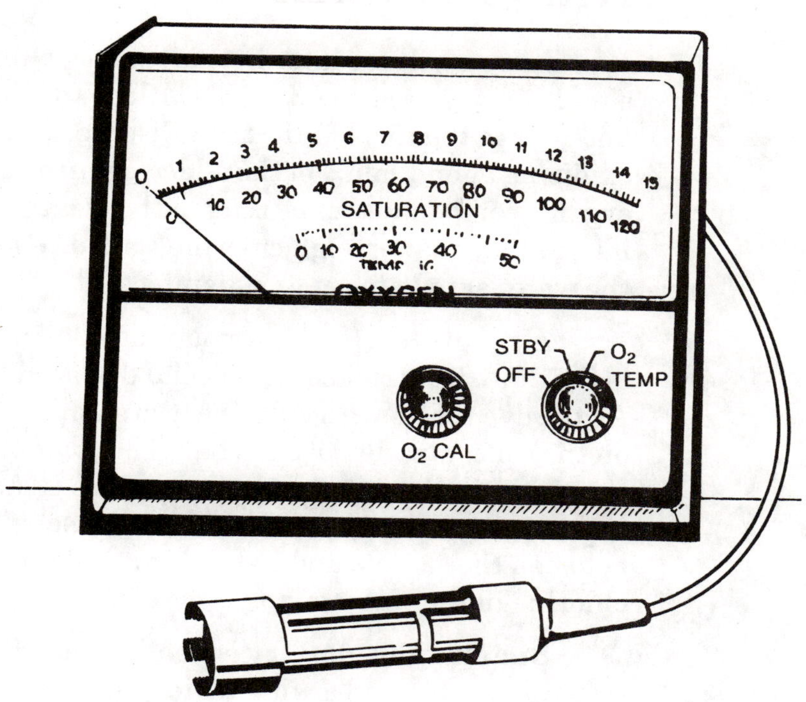

Figure 5-4 Dissolved-oxygen probe

In the Winkler Method of measuring dissolved oxygen, a number of chemical **reagents** are added one step at a time to a water sample. One of these reagents reacts directly with dissolved oxygen in the sample. The product of this first reaction is eventually used to produce free iodine in the water sample. The amount of iodine is directly related to the original amount of dissolved oxygen and can be easily determined by doing a titration. (A titration, you may remember from Subunit 3, involves adding a known concentration of solution to an unknown until an endpoint is reached.)

Testing pH

The pH paper you have used in exercises in this unit is not precise enough to use in water-quality testing. Instead, a pH meter and probe are used to measure the pH of samples to within 0.1 pH unit. Like the dO_2 probe, the pH probe has a pair of electrodes. Before you use a pH meter, it must be **calibrated** by dipping the probe in a buffer solution of known pH and adjusting the pH scale on the meter to agree with the pH of the buffer solution.

Testing for Chlorine

As you will see later in this section, chlorine is added to a water supply during treatment. This is done to destroy bacteria and viruses and reduce the risk of infectious disease. Since chlorine is a strong oxidizing agent, much of the added chlorine quickly combines with organic compounds remaining in the treated water. A chlorine test must verify that enough chlorine, called **residual chlorine**, is left in the water supply to act as a disinfectant.

A simple test for the amount of chlorine present in treated water is the **colorimetric** test. A special dye is added to the water sample. As the dye reacts with chlorine, the sample changes color depending on the concentration of chlorine. The color of the sample after reaction with the dye is compared to a series of standard solutions of dye and varying amounts of chlorine. The technician looks for a match between the sample and a standard to identify the level of residual chlorine in the water supply.

Spectrophotometry is another technique that is also useful for testing chlorine and a wide variety of contaminants in water samples, including:

- Other disinfectants, such as fluorides
- Nutrients, especially nitrates, phosphates, and sulfates
- Metals such as iron, copper, and chromium
- Mineral ions that contribute to water **hardness**, such as calcium and magnesium ions.

In spectrophotometry, a water sample is first treated with a special reagent to produce a color change. Then the treated sample is placed in a device called a spectrophotometer. Inside the spectrophotometer, a given **wavelength** of light is shone through the sample. The meter on the spectrophotometer indicates how much light of the given wavelength the treated sample is absorbing. This reading relates directly to the level of contaminant in the water sample. (The special reagent added is not considered a contaminant for the purposes of the test.)

Test for Biochemical Oxygen Demand (BOD)

Activity 5-8

- Obtain a sample of distilled water, pond water, tap water or other sample provided by your instructor.
- Fill two small bottles to overflowing with the water sample. Tightly stopper the bottles. Label them A and B.
- Place bottle A in a dark incubator at 20°C and do not open for five days.
- Test the dissolved-oxygen level in bottle B using a dissolved-oxygen test kit (or probe). Do not aerate the sample. Record this level in your ABC notebook.
- After five days, test the dO_2 level in bottle A using the dO_2 test kit. Do not aerate the sample. Record this level in your ABC notebook.
- Compare the dO_2 levels from bottles A and B. Explain any difference in dO_2 level.
- Compare your results with groups that tested a different source of water. Explain differences in results between groups.

When microbes are present in water that contains organic matter, the microbes consume dissolved oxygen. Using the oxygen, they break down (oxidize) the organics to obtain energy. The microbial activity is said to place a **biochemical oxygen demand**, or **BOD**, on the water. The BOD is computed by measuring the amount of dO_2 used up by microbes in samples of water over time. The BOD value is thus an indication of the amount of organic material in water.

JOB PROFILE: WASTEWATER TREATMENT TECHNICIAN

Janice C. works in the water-quality lab at the municipal wastewater-treatment plant. One of her daily tasks is to determine the BOD of a sample of wastewater. Janice explains, " First I dilute the sample, usually on the order of 1-5%. Then I pour the sample into each of two bottles until they overflow. Then I tightly stopper both bottles to keep out additional oxygen. One bottle is placed in a dark incubator at 20°C for five days. I keep the other bottle out and determine its dO_2 level using the Winkler Method."

Janice continues, "After five days, I measure the dO_2 in the incubated bottle. The difference in dO_2 levels between the two bottles is related to the amount of dissolved oxygen consumed by microbes in the five-day bottle during the incubation period.

"The BOD test isn't the only test I carry out on the treated wastewater. It is, however, the one to which I must pay most attention, since it can't be completed at one time."

How Is Wastewater Treated?

Figure 5- 5 represents a flow diagram of the wastewater treatment process. **Primary wastewater treatment** involves the separation of colloids and suspended solids from the incoming waste. Separation is done both mechanically and chemically in a multistage process. **Secondary wastewater treatment** accomplishes the final removal of soluble organic substances from the wastewater. It also may include a disinfection step.

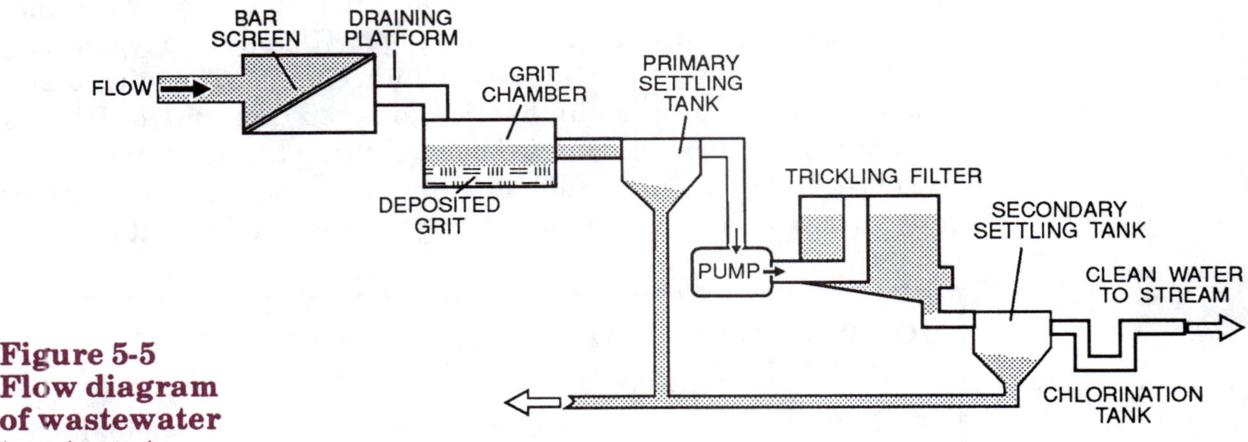

Figure 5-5 Flow diagram of wastewater treatment

A final series of treatments (not shown) might include removal of nitrogen and phosphorous, demineralization, destruction of bacteria and viruses, and removal of organic chemicals and heavy metals remaining after secondary treatment. Such processes that follow secondary treatment are referred to as **tertiary treatment** (meaning third in a sequence), or advanced treatment.

Primary Treatment—Removing Suspended Solids and Colloids

Wastewater entering a treatment plant is first coarsely filtered by screens and other mechanical filters (Figure 5-5). The water is then passed to primary settling basins. During primary treatment the majority of suspended solids and colloids is removed. In the settling basins (Figure 5-5), some of the suspended matter will begin to settle to the bottom due to gravity.

Secondary Treatment—Removing Organics from Wastewater

Primary treatment typically removes about 60% of suspended solids in the original wastewater and about 35% of all organic material contributing to BOD (both suspended and dissolved solids). The organics contributing to the remaining BOD can be further reduced in secondary treatment, generally to about 5% of the original amount.

Secondary treatment involves the biochemical oxidation of organic matter usually in a **trickling filter** (Figure 5-5). This microbial mass has an enormous surface area for the absorption of organic matter. The temperature and chemical composition of the secondary wastewater are kept optimum for the activity of the microbes and a substrate, such as stone, is supplied on which the microbes can grow.

The effluent from the trickling filter enters a settling tank so that solid wastes from the secondary treatment can settle out. These may include by-products of oxidation, dead microbes, and unconsumed organics.

Tertiary or Advanced Treatment

One type of advanced treatment that is infrequently used in wastewater-treatment plants is filtering through **activated carbon**. Molecules of substances remaining in the wastewater adsorb onto the surface of carbon granules. This can greatly improve the quality of water by removing coloring agents, odors, and even such pollutants as herbicides and pesticides. After heavy use, an activated carbon filter can be regenerated by heating it in a furnace at 900°C – 930°C. These high temperatures cause all organic matter adsorbed by the filter to vaporize. The filter is then free to adsorb more pollutant molecules.

Activity 5-9

- Obtain a small amount of activated charcoal on a piece of filter paper. Put the charcoal into a buret (or glass column with rubber hose and pinch clamp). Place a 100-ml beaker or flask below the column to catch the effluent.
- Fill the column with water and release the clamp or open the stopcock until all of the water has run through into the beaker.
- Fill the buret containing the wetted charcoal with dye. Control the flow of effluent with the stopcock or pinch clamp until the effluent is clear.
- Do the experiment again, this time using twice the amount of charcoal in the column and maintaining the flow rate that cleared the effluent most quickly.
- From your results, discuss factors that are important in water filtering.

A chemical process called **coagulation** used for settling of nitrates and phospates in wastewater. In coagulation, a chemical, often alum (aluminum sulfate), is rapidly mixed with the wastewater to help clump together colloidal particles. In a water supply with natural carbonates (water with hardness), the alum reacts in the following way:

$$\underset{\text{alum}}{Al_2(SO_4)_3} + \underset{\text{calcium bicarbonate}}{3Ca(HCO_3)_2} \rightarrow \underset{\text{aluminum hydroxide}}{2Al(OH)_3\downarrow} + \underset{\text{calcium sulfate}}{3CaSO_4} + \underset{\text{carbon dioxide}}{6CO_2}$$

Equation 5-4

The downward arrow after aluminum hydroxide indicates that it forms a precipitate and will therefore be removed from the wastewater through settling. Notice from the equation, however, that there is a trade-off when using chemical coagulants such as alum. What has entered the water supply as a result of the coagulation process? (Refer again to Equation 5-4.)

The wastewater is then slowly stirred so that clusters of solids are formed. The mass of solids is called **floc**. Floc settles to the bottom of the settling basin.

Another type of advanced water treatment takes place outside the treatment plant. It is generally referred to as land treatment. The final effluent from a wastewater-treatment plant is allowed to run off over ground. It is further cleaned as the soil and associated materials filter out remaining pollutants. Because wastewater after secondary treatment contains some nitrogen, phosphorous and organic material, land treatment is useful not only to irrigate but to fertilize dry and nutrient-depleted farmland.

Win, Lose or Compromise

Veronica walks into Ms. Li's class, holding up a newspaper. "Did you see this, Ms. Li?" she asks. "'Council OKs Hondo Springs Ordinance.'"

"They voted on it last night?" Ms. Li asks excitedly. "But which one, the Lopez ordinance or the compromise ordinance?"

"The compromise ordinance," says Leroy. "Well, some people think that anything except no development is a compromise. Councilmember Lopez's ordinance was stricter than the one that passed, but it didn't even get seconded. And Councilmember Carol Overby was the only one to vote against the compromise ordinance, saying it put too many requirements on developers."

"How do you guys feel about the one that passed?" asks Ms. Li.

"Well, I think it wasn't as strict as it could have been, but it's got a lot of water protection in it," answers Veronica.

Leroy agrees. "It surprised me," he says, "I didn't think anybody was really going to listen to the environmental side of this."

"Yeah, they did listen," says Veronica, "but it wasn't easy. It took a whole lot of people. And look how many meetings they went to! There was a lot of pressure."

"And facts," says Ms. Li. "Don't forget, some of those people were informed."

Looking Back

Water can become polluted at different stages of its cycle: evaporation, condensation and precipitation, runoff and percolation. Pollution can be defined as the alteration of the chemical, physical, biological and radiological integrity of the water. There are many types of pollution, including salts, toxic substances, organic wastes, sediment, acids, bacteria and viruses, nutrients, oil and grease, heat and radioactivity.

Water can become polluted through natural processes such as leaching and flooding, through human waste-disposal practices, and through accidental leaks or spills of polluting material.

People who track pollution separate its sources into two groups. Point-source pollution is material discharged directly from a specific source, such as untreated or inadequately treated discharges from an industrial process or a municipal treatment plant. Nonpoint source is harder to identify; it includes storm runoff, leaching agricultural chemicals, and atmospheric contaminants.

Whether point source or nonpoint source, pollution can come from agricultural, industrial or domestic water users. Agricultural users may contaminate water with agrochemicals, salts from irrigation, and animal wastes from feedlot operations. Steam electric power generation also requires a lot of water, but most of the power generating process does not involve polluting chemicals. Some industrial processes are very polluting if wastewater is left untreated. Some of the industries of concern are chemical manufacturing, metals, mining, textiles and paper.

Pollution can be prevented in a variety of ways: halting or limiting the use of polluting chemicals, reducing the water used in a process or use, recycling wastes, treating wastes, storing wastes properly, and preventing leaks and spills of pollutants. These methods can be applied to agricultural, industrial and domestic handling of potential pollutants and uses of water.

Wastewater testing ensures that treatment has been adequate, but it is also used to monitor the treatment processes themselves. At least seven tests are routinely carried out at treatment plants: total solids, organic and inorganic solids, dissolved oxygen, pH, chlorine residual, and biological oxygen demand (BOD).

Treatment of wastewater is divided into three main stages: primary—removal of suspended solids and colloids; secondary—removal or organics; and tertiary—removal of coloring agents, odors and pollutants such as pesticides.

Further Discussion

- The U. S. Environmental Protection Agency carries out research on water-treatment methods and storage, handling and disposal of hazardous chemicals. Contact the E.P.A. to find out what new methods of water treatment are becoming available. Will the water-treatment plant of the future be different from the typical plant of today? If so, how?
- Presently, most of us pay for the water we use if we are taking from a municipal treatment system. However, we are not charged—as individuals or as industries—according to how much we may pollute the water. People who live in rural areas, including most agricultural users, can take the water they need from underground. It may be returned to the water cycle through runoff and percolation in a contaminated state. (Keep in mind that farmers also produce our food supply using the water they take from underground or surface sources.) What kind of system of water use might encourage the prevention of pollution or reduction in water use?

Activities by Occupational Area

General

Water-Quality Regulation at the Local Level

Find out what agency or department of your local government is responsible for handling water-pollution problems. How do they monitor water quality? Are there local water-quality ordinances that they must enforce? How do they work with the state and federal agencies that monitor water quality?

Testing Water Quality

- Contact the Environmental Protection Agency, local civil engineering firm, regional water-quality board or agency, or other organization that hires environmental technicians to test water quality.

- Interview the person who carries out such tests. Find out what tests are used and what aspect of water quality they indicate.

Agriculture and Agribusiness

Agrochemical Producers

Write to some agrochemical producers such as Dupont or Monsanto and ask for information about what new agrochemicals are being produced and how they might be expected to affect water quality, especially as compared with agrochemicals developed in the past.

LISA and Organic Farmers

Interview a farmer in your area who farms "organically" (without the use of agrochemicals) or whose methods fit the name LISA (low-input sustainable agriculture). Find out how they manage to get by with no or fewer agrochemicals, what kinds of crops they grow, what kind of market they target, and how water-use practices differ from those of other farmers.

Health Occupations

Water-Borne Diseases

- Ask different members of the class to investigate different ones of the waterborne diseases listed below:

  - cholera
  - hepatitis
  - infantile diarrhea
  - typhoid fever
  - dysentery
  - polio

- Answer the following questions: What are the causes and symptoms of the disease? Where is this disease common? How many cases of the disease are reported each year in your county? What steps do those in public health occupations take to prevent outbreaks of waterborne diseases? Contact your health department.

- Report your findings to the class.

Home Economics

Reducing Water Pollution from Domestic Sources

- Using the list of ways to prevent pollution given in this subunit, come up with a list of ways that individual users can help to prevent water pollution.
- Make a large display for the list suitable for a school-wide bulletin board and get permission to display it. Make it graphically pleasing and attention-getting.

Industrial Technology

Industrial Waste Reduction

- Write to or arrange to talk with the plant manager of a manufacturing company of your choice. Find out what that company is doing to reduce wastes that may affect wastewater quality.
- Ask about these measures: in-process recycling, using alternative raw materials that do not produce pollutants as products, improving plant operations to reduce leaks and spills, or modifying the production process or the product so that polluting substances are not used.

Treating Wastewater and Drinking Water

- Visit you local water-treatment plant and the sewage-treatment plant.
- Interview the plant manager, operator, or water-quality technician to determine the following:
    - The process by which the water is treated
    - The water-quality tests that are run on the water
    - The standards for each test
- Prepare a diagram or flowchart for each of the treatment processes. Indicate on your diagram where water samples are taken and the acceptable range for the results for each test.
- Compare the two processes and prepare a brief report summarizing your findings.

LAB 10

TESTING WATER QUALITY

PREVIEW

Introduction

Sam C. is self-employed in swimming pool maintenance. He operates his business out of a van, which is filled with pool-cleaning equipment and jugs of pool chemicals.

"My most important job," says Sam, "is making sure the pool water is chemically balanced. To do this I take a small sample of water and run a chemical analysis using a portable test kit. The kit tests for chlorine, pH, alkalinity, water hardness, metals, and a number of other factors.

"Unless some major problem is evident, I start by looking for a chlorine level of about 1.0-1.5 parts per million and a pH slightly on the alkaline side, 7.4-7.6. A high pH can inactivate chlorine and may even cause scaling. Alkalinity is a factor that helps control pH. It should be between 80 and 150 ppm depending on the material from which the pool is made. I may also run tests for metals if staining is evident and for hardness if problems such as scaling are evident.

"If the chlorine test reads low," Sam continues, "I check the pool's chlorinating system. Only the bigger pools, such as those at clubs or city parks actually use a gas-chlorinating system. Home pools generally use a solid form of chlorine. In either case the chlorine must be stabilized with special chemicals. This is because free (unstabilized) chlorine breaks down rapidly in bright sunlight. Solid forms of chlorine generally contain adequate amounts of stabilizer. The solid, either a stick or tablets, slowly dissolves into the water and spreads evenly throughout the pool."

After Sam adjusts the pool's pH and alkalinity with chemicals from the van, he adjusts the chlorine level. He does this by placing stabilized sticks or tablets of chlorine either in the skimmer basket at the side of the pool or, in the case of an automatic chlorinator, in the feeders of the water-recirculating system. If there appears to be a problem with algae growth (green, cloudy water) Sam "shocks" the pool by sprinkling granules of stabilized chlorine directly into the water.

After he is sure the water has been properly conditioned, Sam cleans the pool's filter and skimmer basket and runs the pump for a while. By the time Sam packs up his van to head for lunch, another sick pool is already starting to look healthy again.

Purpose

In this lab, you will test water samples for the presence of dissolved substances.

Lab Objectives

When you've finished this lab, you will be able to—

- Determine whether water is properly chlorinated.
- Make recommendations on how a water supply should be treated based on results of water-quality tests.

Lab Skills

You will use these skills to complete this lab—

- Add reagents drop by drop to a liquid sample.
- Match the color change in a sample to a set of standard colors.

Materials and Equipment Needed

pool and spa test kits for pH, Cl, alkalinity and hardness

bottled water: distilled, deionized, and/or spring water

tap water

swimming-pool or hot-tub water

LAB PROCEDURE

Pre-Lab Discussion

Chlorine is used as a disinfectant in a water supply for a number of reasons. First, it is a strong oxidizing agent; it reacts with the types of organic compounds that make up living cells. (Single-celled organisms such as bacteria and algae are especially vulnerable to chlorine.) Chlorine is also useful because it exists in a number of forms that are water-soluble. One of these is hypochlorite (OCl^-), which is often found as calcium hypochlorite, $Ca(OCl)_2$. Calcium hypochlorite dissolves in water to form hypochlorous acid (HClO) according to the following equation:

$$Ca(OCl)_2 + 2H_2O \rightarrow 2HOCl + Ca^{+2} + 2OH^-$$

In all these forms the chlorine atom is an effective oxidizing agent. A one-time application of chlorine to an outdoor water supply, however, is not likely to remain effective for long. For one thing, an outdoor pool of water constantly receives some input of organic matter. When chlorine reacts with organic compounds it is no longer free to react as a disinfectant. Second, sunlight degrades hypochlorite and some other forms of chlorine. To overcome this latter problem, special organic stabilizers, such as cyanuric acid, are applied during chlorination. Cyanuric acid associates with the chlorine in such a way that chlorine is still available as an oxidizing agent yet is no longer vulnerable to sunlight.

In this lab you will test water from various sources for chlorine level using a colorimetric test. To do the test you collect a water sample and add to it a few drops of a reagent. If chlorine is present the sample will change color. By matching the colored sample against a set of standards of different colors, you can get a good estimate of the level of free (available) chlorine in the sample. If your test kit contains the appropriate reagents and standards, you can do a number of other water-quality tests on the sample.

Safety Precautions

- Do not get test reagents on your skin or clothes, or in your eyes.
- Do not drink water samples either before or after testing.

Method

Part I. Testing a Drinking-Water Supply

Do the following for each test you conduct:

1. Draw water from the tap (or pour bottled water) into the sample vial.

2. Put on your gloves and goggles at this time. Add drops of the appropriate reagent as indicated on the reagent bottle or test kit instructions. Wait for a color change.
3. Match the sample vial to the set of standards. Determine the value for the test.
4. Record test results in Data Table 1.

Data Table 1

Source of Water	Cl (ppm)	pH	Hardness (ppm)	Alkalinity (ppm)
A. Tap water				
B. Bottled water:				
Distilled				
Deionized				
Spring				

Part II. Testing Water from Swimming Pools, Hot Tubs, etc.

Do the following for each test you conduct:

1. Collect water in the sample vial by immersing the vial at least 18" below the surface of the pool.

2. Put on your gloves and goggles at this time. Add drops of the appropriate reagent as indicated on the reagent bottle or test kit instructions. Wait for a color change.
3. Match the sample vial to the set of standards. Determine the value for the test.
4. Record test results in Data Table 2.

Data Table 2

Pool or Spa Tested	1. _____	2. _____
Pool dimensions*	ℓ = — $d^{\dagger}$ = — w = — *dia* = —	ℓ = — $d^{\dagger}$ = — w = — *dia* = —
Type and frequency of chlorination		
Cl (ppm)		
pH		
Hardness (ppm)		
Alkalinity (ppm)		

* Use maximum length and width for oval pool; record only diameter and depth for round pool.

† Estimate average depth of pool.

Cleanup Instructions

- Dispose of water samples into the drain.
- Rinse vials with distilled water before returning to kits.
- Make sure all reagent bottles are tightly capped.

WRAP-UP

Conclusions

1. Explain the results of your tests in Part I.
   - What do the values for chlorine, pH, alkalinity, and hardness indicate about the water you tested?
   - Compare the results of your tests on tap versus bottled water. From which source of water would you prefer to drink, and why?
2. Explain the results of your tests in Part II.
   - What do the values for chlorine, pH, alkalinity, and hardness indicate about the operating condition of the pool or spa from which you drew your sample?
   - If the test results do not fall in the desirable range, what steps would you take to chemically balance the pool?

Challenge Questions and Extensions

3. You have been asked by a customer to reopen a home swimming pool that you drained the previous fall. The pool has an automatic chlorinator system that uses stabilized chlorine cartridges. The cartridge manufacturer recommends adding a 1-ounce cartridge of stabilized chlorine per thousand gallons of water at 80-90°F.
   - You have just filled the pool with city water and checked to be sure all your mechanical equipment is clean and operating correctly. What must you do next to decide the right size chlorine cartridge for the chlorination system?
   - For a pool you or your lab partner sampled in Part II of the Method, which size chlorine cartridge should be used? (Assume water temperature of 80-90°F.) Get help from your teacher in determining the number of gallons of water a pool of your dimensions holds at full capacity.
4. For each pool or spa problem in the table below, investigate the most likely cause(s) of the problem and treatments for the problem based on the cause.

Problem	Most Likely Cause(s)	Recommended Treatment
Foaming		
Stains on walls		
Scaling on walls and in water lines		
Cloudy water		
Colored water		
Complaints about skin or eye irritation		

UNIT WRAP-UP ACTIVITY

Throughout this unit, you have done several activities that involved gathering different kinds of data from an aquatic habitat. You gathered physical data and chemical data, and surveyed the plant and animal life in and around the habitat. Prepare a three- to five-minute presentation of your data and give it in front of your class. The presentation should include your data and your conclusions about the state of the ecology in the habitat; that is, are the animal and plant life forms in it healthy or dying out. Are there any problems with the habitat that your data can identify? Support your conclusions with your data.

As each person presents his or her data, compile the data on the chalkboard in a table similar to the one below. If any of the habitat areas are along the same stream, or in different parts of the same lake, or connected in other ways, compare the data for these connected habitats to see if there are similarities in the data.

After everyone has presented his or her data, discuss as a class the health of your local aquatic habitats. Are there problems that you can identify from the data? Discuss possible solutions to any problems you identify.

Data Table

Location	Air Temperature	Water Temperature	pH	Dissolved Oxygen
Location	**Survey of Life Forms**			

GLOSSARY

acid rain – rain that has a pH equal to or less than 5

acid-base neutralization – said of a chemical reaction in which the amounts of acid and base react to form water (and salt) and leave no excess of H_3O^+ or OH^- ions. The resulting solution has a pH of 7.

activated carbon – a highly adsorbent form of carbon used to remove contaminants from fluids

agrochemicals – commercial chemicals used in agriculture, such as livestock hormones, fertilizers, herbicides, and pesticides

alkaline – having a pH greater than 7, basic

anion – any atom or group of atoms with a negative charge

aquifer – underground rock formation that contains water

bases – substances that, when mixed with water, form hydroxide ions

biochemical oxygen demand (BOD) – the amount of oxygen required to oxidize a given amount of organic material

calibrate – to check, adjust, or standardize the graduations of a measuring instrument

catalyst – any substance that increases the rate of a chemical reaction but is not altered in the reaction

cation – any atom or group of atoms with a positive charge

chemical equilibrium – the condition in a chemical reaction in which the reactants are converting to products at the same rate that the products are converting back to reactants

coagulation – the formation of a liquid into a semisolid or solid mass

colligative properties – properties such as vapor pressure and freezing point that are determined by the number of solute particles in a solution rather than by the chemical properties of the solute

colloidal suspensions – small particles in a liquid that are kept permanently suspended

colorimetric test – a method of chemical analysis in which the color of a solution is compared to standard colors representing known values

concentration – number of molecules or atoms of a substance relative to the space that the substance occupies

condense – to change from gaseous state to liquid state; such as, when water vapor condenses to form water

conduction – the process in which heat energy flows from an area of higher temperature to an area of lower temperature

density – mass per unit volume of a substance

diffusion – random movement of molecules of a dissolved or suspended substance due to the energy of the molecules themselves

dilute – said of a solution with a small amount of solute; to make a solution less concentrated by adding additional solvent

dissolved oxygen concentration (dO_2) – the amount of oxygen gas (O_2) dissolved in water, usually measured in milligrams per liter of water or parts per million of oxygen to water

dissolving – the process of forming a mixture of 2 or more substances that is the same throughout. One component of the mixture is the solvent and there is more solvent in the mixture than any other component. The other components of the mixture are called the solute and can be solid, liquid, or gas.

electrodes – terminals that conduct electric current or that emit, collect, or control the flow of electrons

empirical formula – the simple ratio of the number of atoms of elements in the compound

emulsion – suspension of one liquid in another liquid

enzymes – specialized protein molecules that speed up the rate of chemical reactions

equivalent – the weight of solute that will supply one mole of reacting material in a solution

eutrophication – a part of the normal aging process of lakes in which they become enriched with nutrients, and silt and organic matter settle out, filling them up

fertilizer – a substance added to soil to supplement its nutrient content

floc – a fluffy mass formed by the clustering of suspended particles

food pyramid – a graphic representation of a biological community in terms of the numbers of organisms present (or their total mass or value in calories)

groundwater – water that is found below Earth's surface

guard cells – pairs of cells that control the opening and closing of pores (stomata) leading to the internal tissues of the plant

habitat – the physical environment in which an organism lives

hardness – the amount of a salt, usually calcium carbonate, dissolved in water

heat of vaporization – the amount of heat required to change one gram of liquid into vapor

homogeneous – said of a mixture that is the same throughout

hydronium ion (H_3O^+) – a cation formed when water ionizes or when acids are added to water

hydroxide ion (OH^-) – an anion formed when water ionizes or when bases are added to water

hypothalamus – a gland at the base of the brain that sends messages to other endocrine glands; functions in the maintaining of constant internal body conditions

in-process recycling – removing waste materials at a particular point in an industrial process and returning them for use somewhere in that process

ions – particles that carry a positive or negative charge. An ion is formed when an atom or a group of atoms gains or loses electrons.

ionization of water – the dissociation of some molecules in a sample of water into H_3O^+ and OH^- ions

kidney – an organ in vertebrate animals that functions to maintain proper water balance, regulate acid-base concentration, and excrete soluble wastes as urine

laser technology – the study of lasers, the electronic devices which control lasers, and the optical systems which focus and shape the laser's light

leaching – process by which water carries dissolved or suspended materials as it percolates down to groundwater

liquid – a phase of matter with a definite volume but no definite shape

logarithm – the exponent that indicates the power to which a number has been raised to produce a given number; $\log_{10} 100 = 2$, since $10^2 = 100$

lymphatic system – an open circulatory system that gathers excess fluid from the body and drains it into the veins of the cardiovascular system

micelles – spheres with the nonpolar tails of molecules pointed to the inside of the sphere and with the charged heads of molecules on the surface

microorganisms (microbes) – single-celled organisms too small to be seen by the naked eye such as bacteria, yeast, algae, protozoans, plankton and viruses

molar concentration – the number of moles per liter of solution

molecular formula – the number of each type of atom in a molecule of a compound

negative logarithm – a notation which gives the logarithm ($\log_{10}$) of a number between 1 and 0 a positive value

neutral – a solution in which the concentrations of positive and negative ions are equal; a compound that is neither alkaline nor acidic

neutral solution – any solution in which the H_3O^+ and OH^- ion concentrations are equal

nonpolar – said of a molecule having no separation of charges, or having a symmetry of charges about the center of the molecule

normality – the number of equivalents of solute per liter of solution

osmosis – diffusion of water across a selectively permeable membrane, from an area of greater water concentration to an area of lesser water concentration

overdraft – groundwater withdrawn over a period of time at a faster rate than it can be replenished

percent composition – the most common way of expressing concentration, either as percent by weight (solids) or percent by volume (liquids)

percent by weight – weight expressed as the mass in grams of solid solute per 100 grams of solution

percent by volume – weight expressed as the volume in milliliters of a liquid solute in 100 milliliters of solution

persistent – remaining fixed in a specific condition or position; said of a substance that remains unchanged and is not broken down or degraded in the environment

pesticide – any substance that kills pests or inhibits their reproduction

phases of matter – one of three states (solid, liquid, or gas) in which most matter can exist

pH scale – a system that indicates the acidity or alkalinity of a solution. Scale values range from 0 to 14.

plankton – microscopic plant-like or animal-like organisms that float or drift in great numbers near the surface of fresh or salt waters

pOH – the negative logarithm of the hydroxide ion concentration in a solution

polar – said of a molecule having a separation of charges resulting in a positive and a negative region of the molecule

polarity of water – property of water responsible for the bonding of water molecules to one another; the negative end of one water molecule is attracted to the positive end of another water molecule

precipitation – any liquid or solid form of water particles that fall from the atmosphere to the ground. Rain, snow, sleet and hail are forms of precipitation.

primary wastewater treatment – steps in the treatment of sewage to remove colloids and suspended solids from wastewater

reagent – a substance used in a chemical reaction to detect, measure, or produce other substances

recharge zone – the land above an aquifer through which water seeps to the aquifer

residual chlorine – the amount of chlorine remaining in water at some time after the water was chlorinated

runoff – water that flows over land after rainfall, snowmelt, or irrigation

saltwater intrusion – displacement of fresh water, either surface or ground water, with salt water as a result of the difference in density

secondary wastewater treatment – sewage treatment done following primary treatment to remove dissolved organic material

sediment – any solid material that settles out of a solution

self-ionization of water – the dissociation of some molecules in a sample of water into H_3O^+ and OH^- ions

solid – a phase of matter with a definite volume and shape

solute – the molecules of the substance that is being dissolved

solutions – mixtures in which one substance (the solute) is being dissolved and the other substance is the dissolving medium (the solvent)

solvent – a substance that can dissolve another substance

spectrophotometry – a method of analyzing a chemical sample based on the amount of light of different wavelengths it absorbs

spontaneously – occurring without the help of an external agent

stomata – the tiny pores in the surface of a leaf or stem through which gases (including water vapor) are absorbed or released

structural formula – the number of atoms of each element and their arrangement in the molecule of a substance

subsidence – sinking of a part of Earth's crust due to removal of underground materials

surface water – water that is visible on Earth's surface

suspensions – a mixture of solid particles in water that are larger than water molecules and tend to settle out

temperature conformers – organisms whose internal temperature fluctuates with changes in environmental temperature

tertiary treatment – any of various methods used to further purify water or wastewater that has already gone through secondary treatment

titration – the process of determining the measured amount of a solution that reacts with a sample

transpiration – the evaporation of water from plant tissues into the surrounding atmosphere

trickling filter – wastewater treatment unit in which microbes absorb and break down organic matter during secondary treatment

volatilize – to evaporate or cause to evaporate

water balance – the difference between water gains by an organism (inputs) and water losses from the organism (outputs) over a specified time period. An organism is said to maintain water balance when water inputs equal water outputs.

water cycle – the process by which water moves through the environment, including rainfall, runoff, seepage, and various forms of evaporation

watershed – the total drainage area where water flows to a common point, such as a creek or lake

water solubility – the ability of a substance to dissolve in water

water vapor – water in the gas phase

wavelength – the distance between two energy peaks of adjacent energy waves. Light is energy radiating within a particular range of wavelengths.

Winkler method – a chemical method used to determine the concentration of dissolved oxygen in a water sample